The Rheumatological Physical Examination

The Rheumatological Physical Examination

Edited by

Hugh Little, M.D.

Head
Division of Rheumatology
Sunnybrook Medical Centre
Toronto, Ontario, Canada

G&S

Grune & Stratton, Inc.
Harcourt Brace Jovanovich, Publishers
Orlando New York San Diego Boston London
San Francisco Tokyo Sydney Toronto

Grune & Stratton, Inc.
Orlando, Florida 32887

Distributed in the United Kingdom by
Grune & Stratton, Ltd.
24/28 Oval Road, London NW 1

Library of Congress Catalog Number 86-9769
International Standard Book Number 0-8089-1824-9
Printed in the United States of America
86 87 88 89 10 9 8 7 6 5 4 3 2 1

Contents

Introduction vii

Contributors ix

1. The Normal Joint 1

2. The Physical Examination of the Normal Joint 9

3. The Abnormal Joint 29

4. The Temporomandibular Joint 37
Jack L. Stein

5. The Neck and Back 43
Hugh Little

6. The Shoulder Girdle 59
Joseph B. Houpt

7. The Shoulder 65
Joseph B. Houpt

8. The Elbow 73
Abraham Chaiton

9. The Radioulnar Joints 79
M. Lynn Russell

10. The Wrist 83
Robert Y. McMurtry

11. The Hand 91
Robert Y. McMurtry

12. The Pelvic Girdle 101
Donald McGillivray

13. The Hip 105
Frances Y-K Leung

14. The Knee 111
Arthur Bookman

15. The Ankle and Foot 121
Adel G. Fam

16. Stance and Gait 131
Gordon Hunter

17. Measurement of Muscle Strength 139
Antoine Helewa

Reading List 145

Index 147

Introduction

Rheumatology is a bedside activity. It is the physical examination that provides most of the information necessary for the diagnosis and management of rheumatological problems.

Abnormalities are suspected from the history, recognized by inspection, and confirmed by palpation. The skills are simple. The interpretation of the findings is difficult and requires an understanding of musculoskeletal development, functional anatomy, and pathological processes.

The trainee in Rheumatology has difficulties to overcome. Too often, the medical undergraduate is trained in a hospital setting where patients are severely ill or have major deformities. These patients present problems that may be overwhelming for the beginner and the common mild musculoskeletal diseases of the ambulatory patient may never be encountered. The postgraduate trainee can become so involved in the search for the cause and cure of rheumatic disease that fundamental bedside facts may be forgotten. To overcome these difficulties the trainee must learn and practice a systematic examination.

Many health disciplines examine the musculoskeletal system. Each discipline has a slightly different interest related to the therapeutic interventions commonly undertaken. Thus, the Orthopedist searches for signs of damage and measures alignment. Physiotherapists measure muscle strength and stamina and the range of motion of joints. Occupational Therapists use functional assessments and students of biomechanics study centers of motion, muscle forces, and lever arms.

The rheumatological examination addresses the questions, "Are the joints normal or abnormal?" If abnormal, "What is the distribution of the abnormality and is the abnormality due to faulty development, inflammation or damage?"

This book describes a system for the physical examination of the rheumatological patient and illustrates the clinical findings upon which the practice of rheumatology is based. It is directed to those who will be examining patients with rheumatological problems. We believe that it will be most useful for the trainee in Rheumatology and for the medical student and intern when doing their Rheumatology rotation. We hope that other disciplines will find it helpful as well.

Chapter 1 is a brief and basic description of the properties of the normal joint. These properties are referred to in the regional chapters.

Chapter 2 describes the 3 minute examination of the normal cooperative patient. Every practicing Rheumatologist has developed a personal variation of this quick, complete examination. It demonstrates the presence and the distribution of joint abnormalities and gives some hints as to their nature.

Chapter 3 describes the abnormal joint and the physical findings that differentiate inflammation from damage.

Chapters 4–15 describe the development, functional anatomy, and physical examination of each joint region. The regional physical examination retraces the steps outlined in Chapters 2 and 3. The regional chapters will be more meaningful if Chapters 2 and 3 are read first.

This text does not address disease entities, their differential diagnosis, or their diagnostic physical signs. Although some clinical conditions such as rheumatoid arthritis and degenerative joint disease are mentioned, they are not described. A full discussion of differential diagnosis and disease entities can be found in the textbooks of Rheumatology in the Reading List.

ACKNOWLEDGMENTS

Rheumatology at the University of Toronto has always placed great emphasis on clinical skills. The late Doctors Wallace Graham, Metro Ogryzlo, and Philip Rosen set a high standard of physical diagnosis. We hope that their standard will be reflected in this volume.

Dr. Hugh Smythe has created a climate of interest in physical examination in Toronto by constantly questioning his associates and trainees on the significance and the technique of their physical findings. He made many of the clinical observations contained in this book. We acknowledge our debt with thanks.

We wish to thank Drs. Michael Aubrey, Philip Baer, Mary Bell, John Dickson, Robert Ikeman, Perry Rush, Jim Main, and John Thompson, who were kind enough to review the manuscript and make many helpful suggestions. We would also like to thank Ellen Hoy for her assistance with the manuscript and Jim Atkinson of the Health Science Media Service at Sunnybrook Medical Centre for his help with the illustrations.

Contributors

Arthur Bookman M.D. (Toronto), F.R.C.P.C.
Rheumatologist
Head
Division of Rheumatology
Toronto General Hospital
101 College Street
Toronto, M5G 1L7 Canada

Abraham Chaiton M.D. (Toronto), F.R.C.P.C.
Rheumatologist
Sunnybrook Medical Centre and
York Finch Hospital
2075 Bayview Avenue
Toronto, M4N 3M5, Canada

Adel Fam M.D. (Cairo), M.R.C.P., F.R.C.P.C.
Rheumatologist
Sunnybrook Hospital
2075 Bayview Avenue
Toronto, M4N 3M5, Canada

Antoine Helewa M.Sc. (McMaster)
Physiotherapist
Chairman
Department of Physical Therapy
Elborn College
University of Western Ontario
London, N6G 1H1, Ontario, Canada

Joseph Houpt M.D. (Toronto) F.R.C.P.C.
Rheumatologist
Head
Division of Rheumatology
Mount Sinai Hospital
600 University Avenue
Toronto, M5G 1B2 Canada

Gordon Hunter M.R.C.S., L.R.C.P., F.R.C.S. (England), F.R.C.S.C.
Orthopedist
Director
Aids for Living Rehabilitation Centre
Sunnybrook Medical Centre
2075 Bayview Avenue
Toronto, M4N 3M5, Canada

Frances Y-K Leung M.D. (Edmonton) F.R.C.P.C.
Rheumatologist
Sunnybrook Medical Centre
2075 Bayview Avenue
Toronto, M4N 3M5, Canada

Hugh Little M.D. (Toronto) F.R.C.P.C.
Rheumatologist
Head
Division of Rheumatology
Sunnybrook Medical Centre
2075 Bayview Avenue
Toronto, M4N 3M5, Canada

Donald McGillivray M.D. (Toronto) F.R.C.P.C.
Rheumatologist
North York Hospital and
Sunnybrook Medical Centre
2075 Bayview Avenue
Toronto, M4N 3M5, Canada

Robert McMurtry M.D. (Toronto) F.R.C.S.C.
Orthopedist
Director
Regional Trauma Unit
Sunnybrook Medical Centre
2075 Bayview Avenue
Toronto, M4N 3M5, Canada

Lynn Russell M.D. (McGill) F.R.C.P.C.
Rheumatologist
Head
Division of Rheumatology
Women's College Hospital
76 Grenville Street
Toronto, M5S 1B2 Canada

Kate Santos D.V.M. (Madrid) B.Sc.A.A.M. (Toronto)
Medical Illustrator
Health Science Media Service
Sunnybrook Medical Centre
2075 Bayview Avenue
Toronto, M4N 3M5, Canada

Jack Stein M.D. (Toronto) F.R.C.P.C.
Rheumatologist
Scarborough General Hospital and
Sunnybrook Medical Centre
2075 Bayview Avenue
Toronto, M4N 3M5, Canada

1
The Normal Joint

CONTROLLED MOBILITY

Joints are discontinuities in the skeleton that allow bones to move on one another. This mobility is controlled by the shape of the articular surfaces, the joint capsule, surrounding ligaments, and by other adjacent structures. Articular cartilage and synovial fluid permit movement to be virtually free of friction. Muscles and their tendons provide the power to resist gravity and to perform purposeful actions.

Each joint needs to be understood in terms of mobility, control, and function.

THE RHEUMATOLOGICAL PHYSICAL EXAMINATION
ISBN 0-8089-1824-9

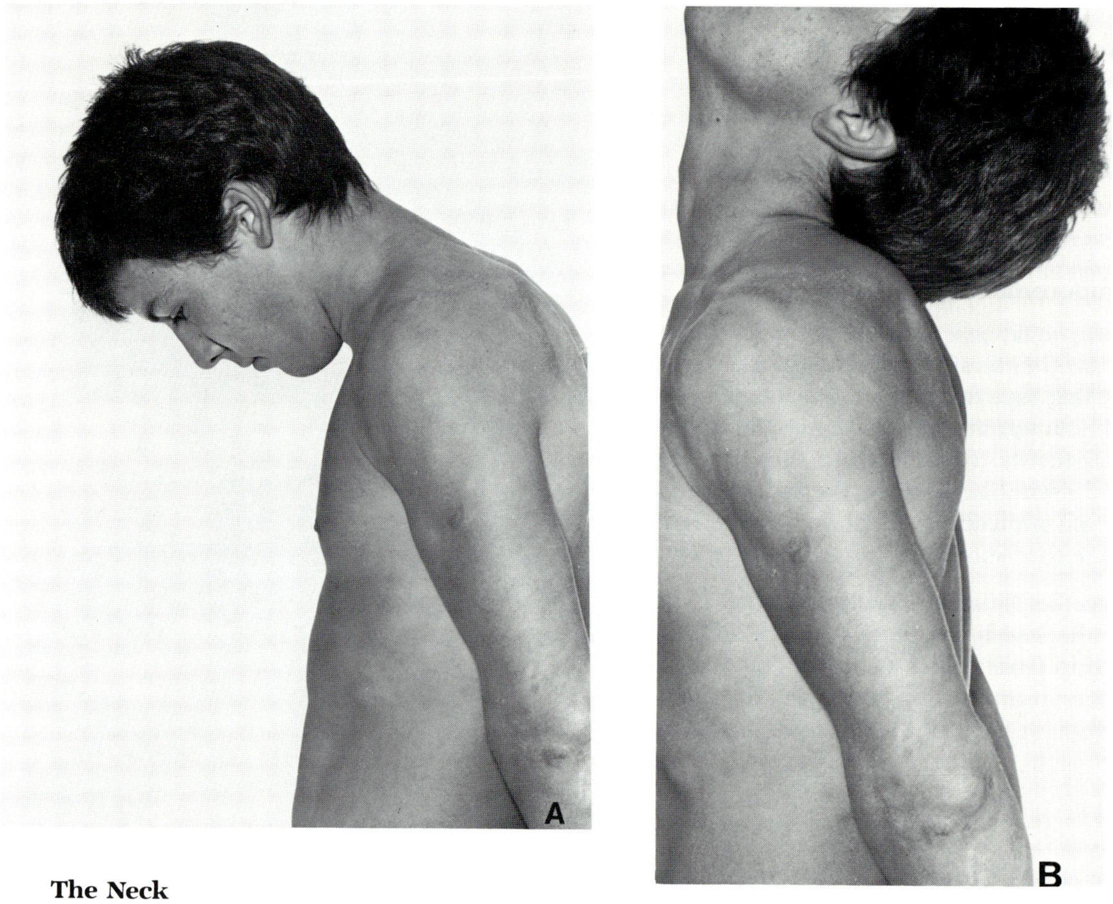

The Neck

Figure 3. (A) Cervical and upper thoracic flexion. (B) Cervical and upper thoracic extension.

Figure 3

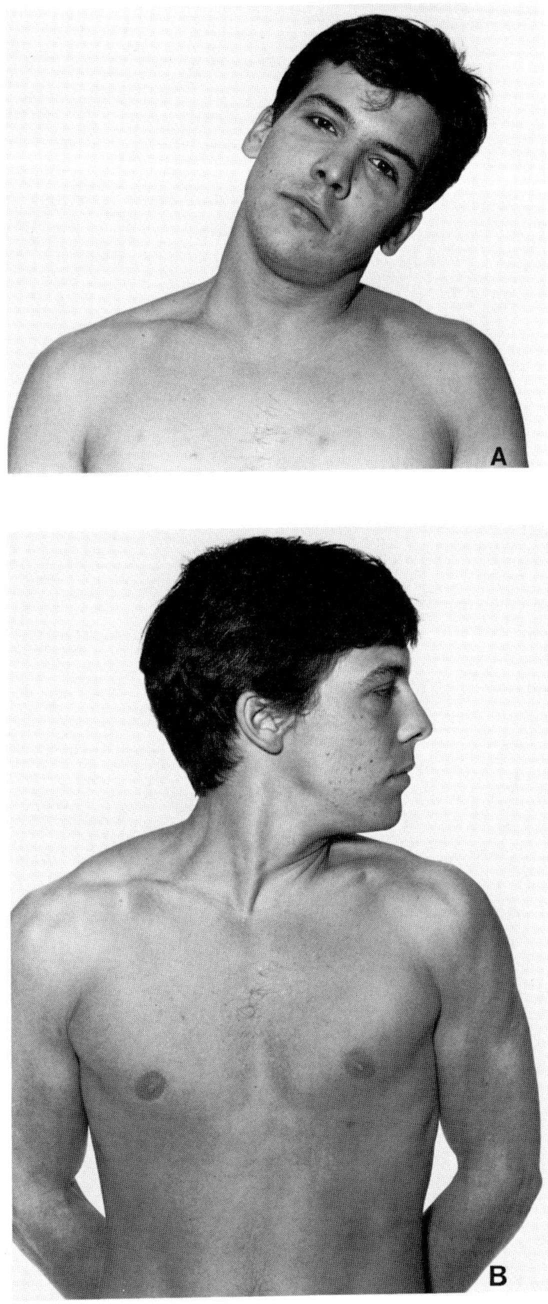

Figure 4

Figure 4. (A) Cervical lateral flexion. (B) Cervical rotation.

The only visible landmark of the cervical spine is the spinous process of C7, thus observations are limited to the spatial relationships of the head and the trunk. In the upright position, the head should be balanced in the midline above the thorax. Movement occurs in three directions, flexion/extension, lateral flexion and rotation. Rotation and lateral flexion are increased if the neck is slightly flexed and the facet joints are partly disengaged.

Some of the range of movement illustrated in the photographs is due to motion of the head on the neck and motion in the upper thoracic spine.

The Shoulder Girdle

Figure 5. The shoulder shrug.

The patient stands facing the examiner with the arms hanging loosely and shrugs the shoulders as high as possible. This demonstrates movement of the shoulder girdle over the chest wall and requires movement at both the sternoclavicular and acromioclavicular joints. The shoulder girdle can also move forward and back on the thorax (not shown).

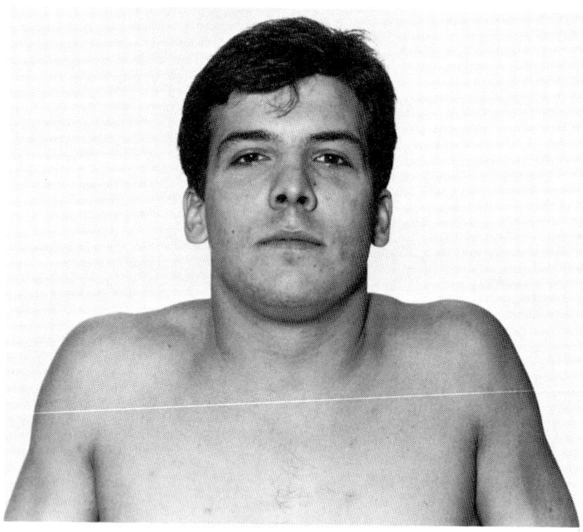

Figure 5

The Shoulder

Figure 6. Total shoulder elevation.

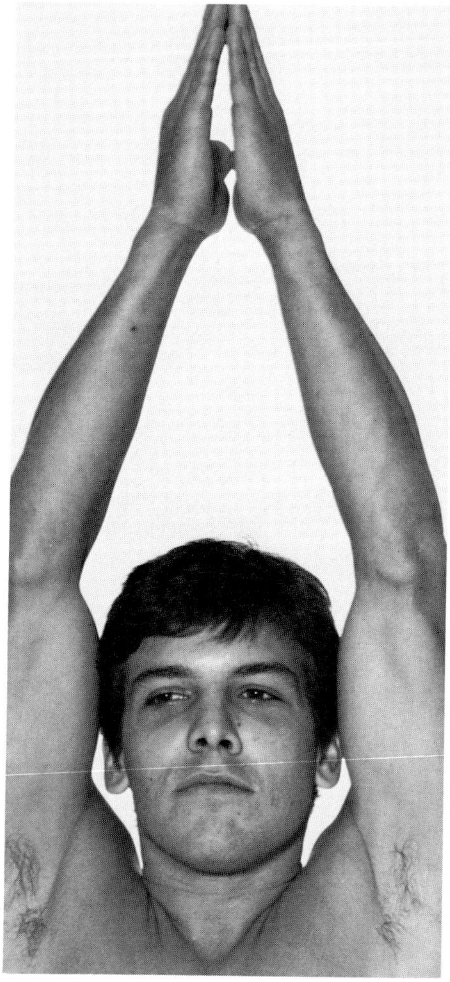

Figure 6

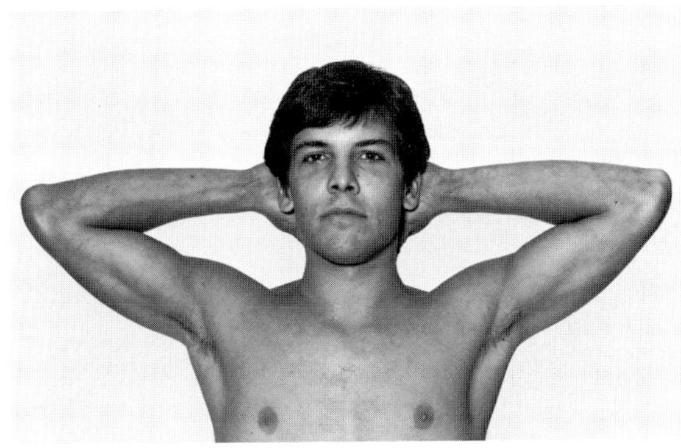

Figure 7

Figure 7. External rotation.
Figure 8. Internal rotation.

The patient elevates the arms to the vertical position. The hands are then placed behind the neck and the elbows moved back until the arms are in the coronal plane. This position demonstrates full external rotation of the shoulder. The arms are then placed behind the back to demonstrate internal rotation.

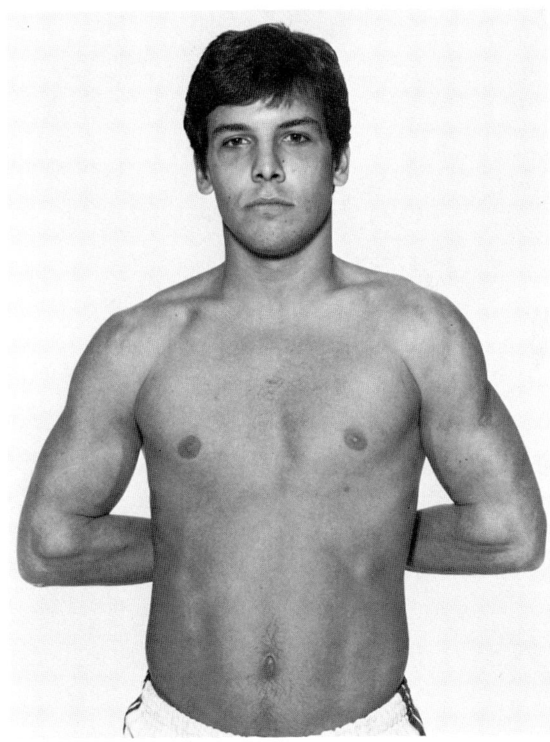

Figure 8

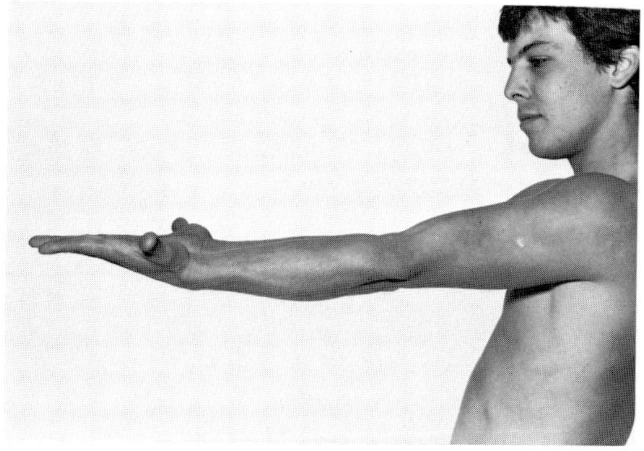

Figure 9

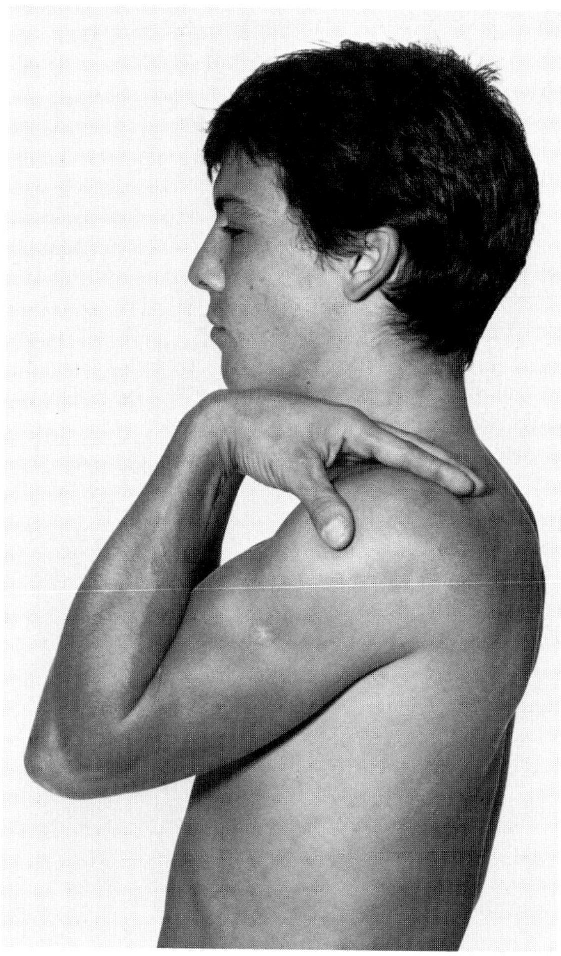

Figure 10

The Elbow

Figure 9. Elbow extension.
Figure 10. Elbow flexion.

The arms are stretched forward with the palm up and the elbow fully extended. The arm and forearm usually form a straight line although muscular people may lack a few degrees and more supple individuals may extend an extra ten degrees. The patient touches the shoulders to demonstrate flexion.

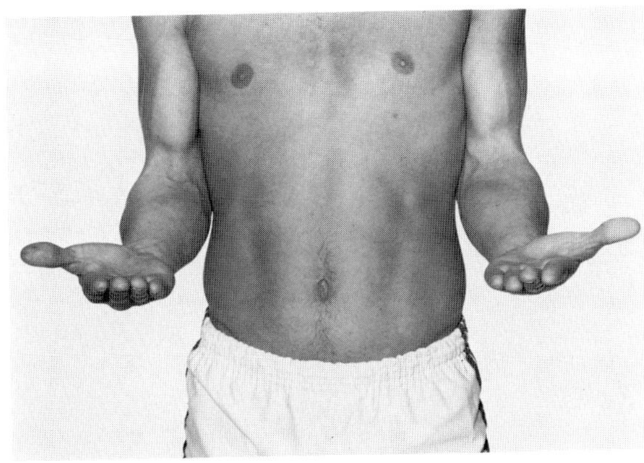

Figure 11

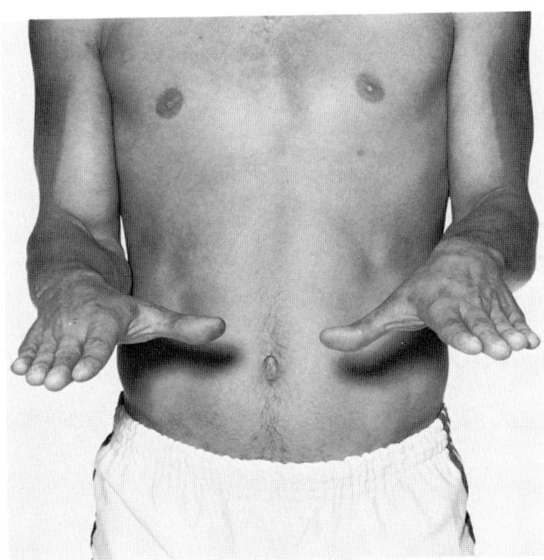

Figure 12

The Radioulnar Joints

Figure 11. Forearm supination.
Figure 12. Forearm pronation.

The arm is held at the side with the elbow bent to 90 degrees to prevent rotation at the shoulder. The hands are fully supinated (turned up) so that the palm is nearly horizontal. Then the hands are fully pronated (turned down) so that the palm is nearly horizontal.

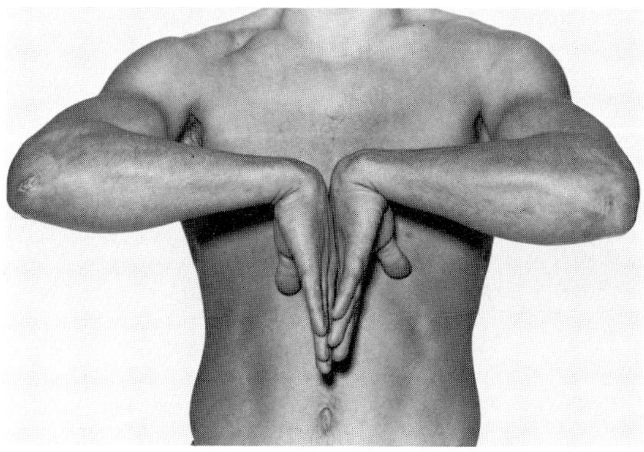

Figure 13

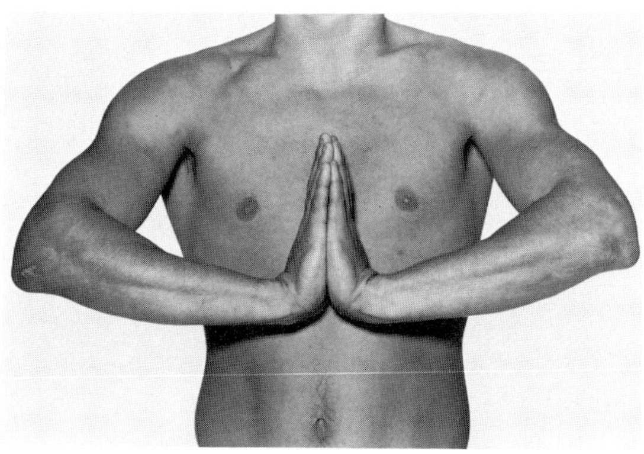

Figure 14

The Wrist

Figure 13. Wrist flexion.
Figure 14. Wrist extension.

With the forearms horizontal, the patient is asked to press the backs of the hands and then the palms of the hands together. This manoeuvre demonstrates a range of movement of over 90 degrees in each direction due to the pressure exerted through the joints. Simple active movement has a smaller range.

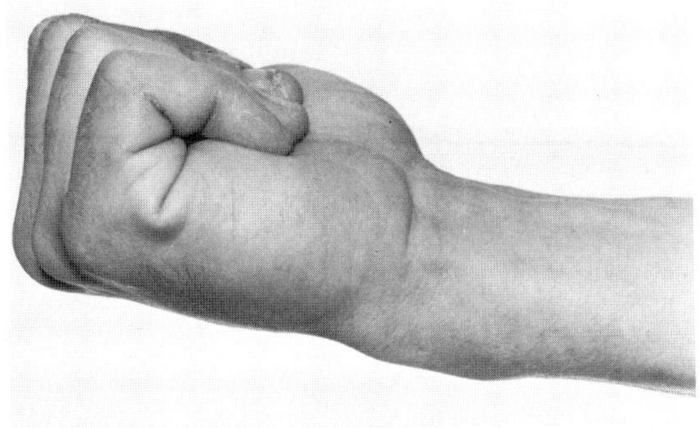

Figure 15

The Hand

Figure 15. Metacarpophalangeal flexion.

Figure 16. Interphalangeal flexion.

Flexion of the metacarpophalangeal joints can be demonstrated by having the patient bring the finger tips to the base of the hand. The patient is then asked to bring the tips of the fingers to the metacarpal eminences to demonstrate flexion at the interphalangeal joints.

Figure 17. Thumb opposition.

With the hand open, the tip of the thumb is then placed on the fifth metacarpal eminence to demonstrate flexion at the carpometacarpal, metacarpophalangeal, and interphalangeal joints.

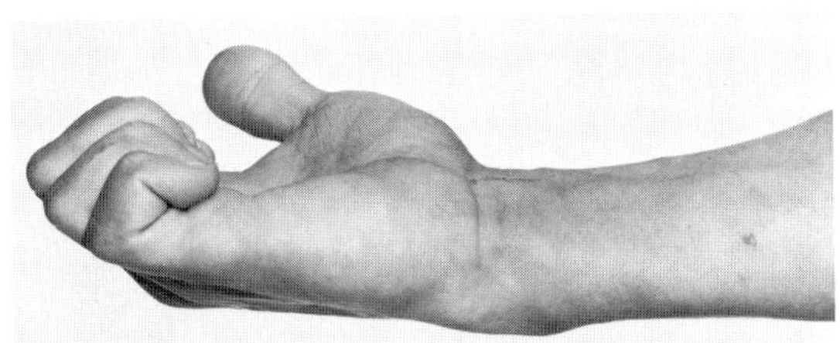

Figure 16

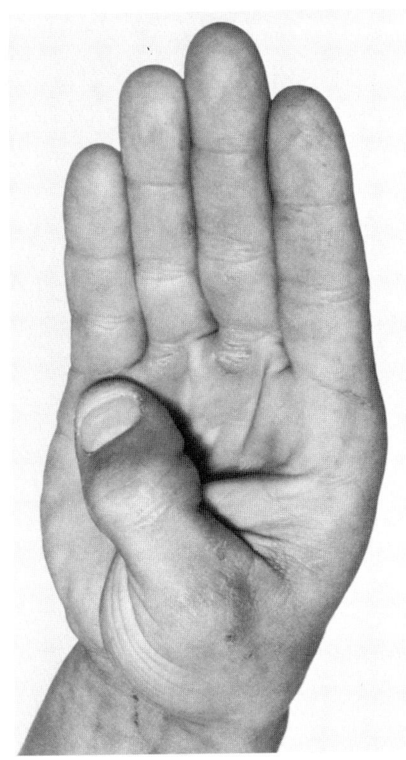

Figure 17

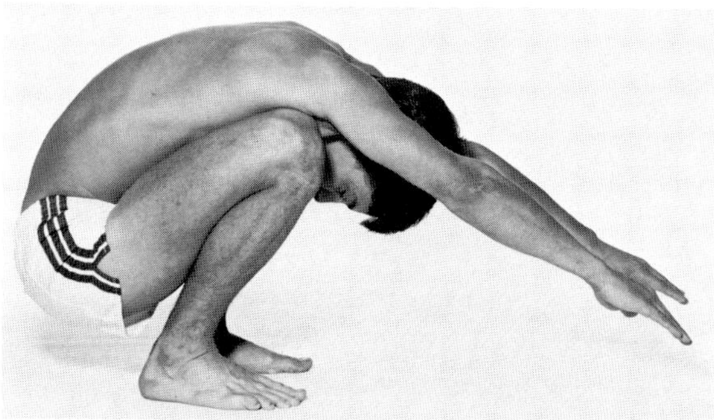

Figure 18

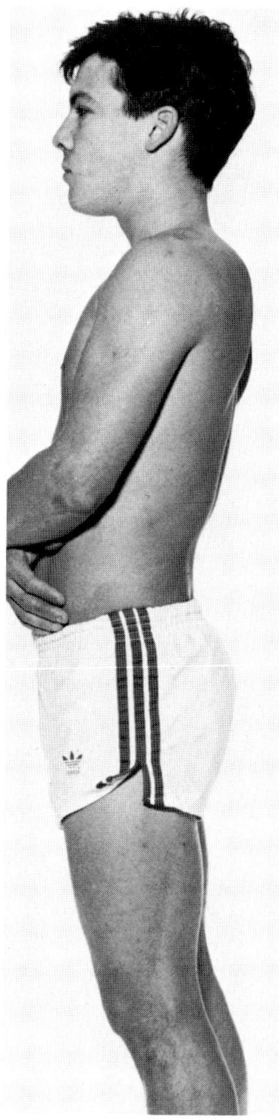

Figure 19

The Back

Figure 18. Full sagittal flexion.
Figure 19. Normal erect position.

Flexion/Extension

In the fully flexed posture the thoraco-lumbar spine forms a smooth curve from the sacrum to the vertebra prominens (C7). The erect position shows the normal thoracic kyphosis and the normal lumbar and cervical lordosis.

Lateral flexion

Figure 20. Spinal lateral flexion.

The normal person can touch the top of the fibula by lateral flexion of the thoracolumbar spine while standing with the feet together and both heels on the ground. The patient needs to be cautioned not to bend forward. Figure 20 illustrates the smooth normal curve from the sacrum to the vertebra prominens.

Rotation

Figure 21. Spinal rotation.

Rotation can be tested in the standing or sitting position. The pelvis is fixed by the examiners hands when standing or it is settled firmly on the chair in the sitting position. The arms are folded across the chest to partially immobilize the shoulder girdle. A plane through the angles of the scapula is compared to a similar plane through the posterior iliac spines. The patient rotates the thorax as far as possible in each direction and the difference between these two planes is estimated in degrees.

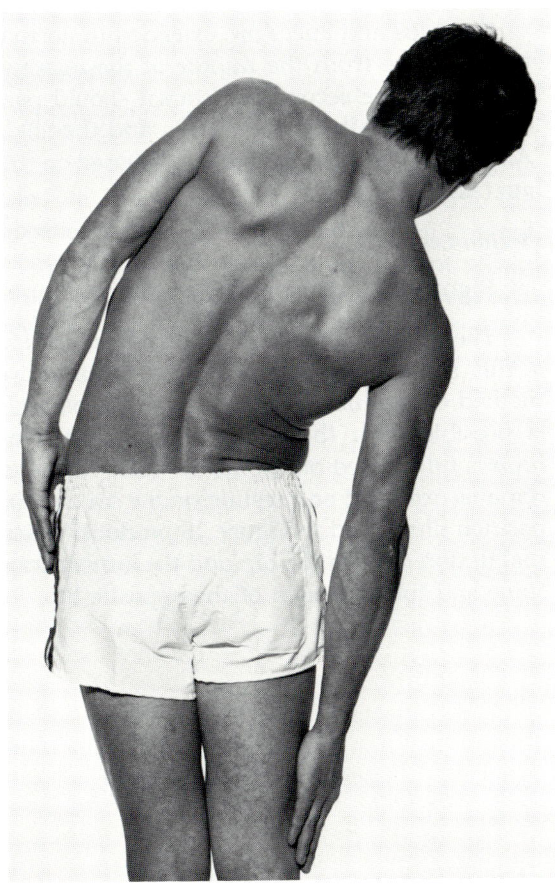

Figure 20

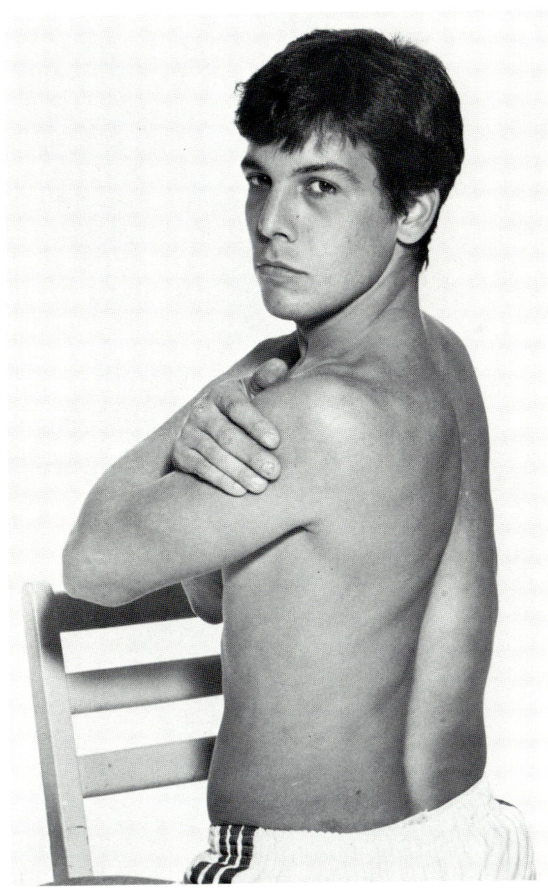

Figure 21

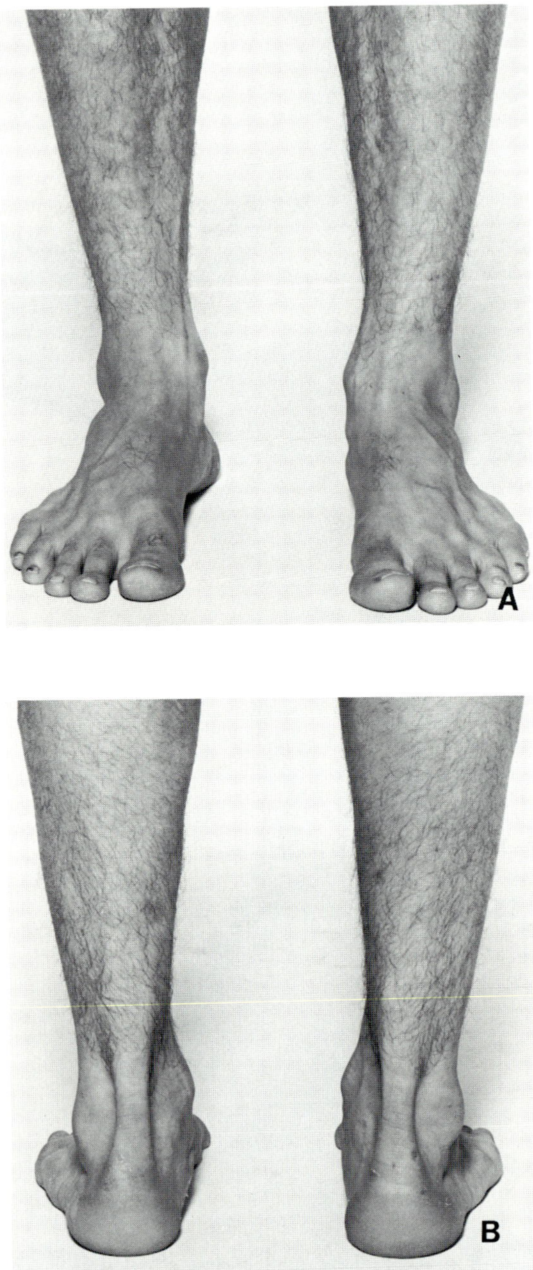

Figure 25

The Ankle

Figure 25. (A&B) Alignment of the ankle and foot.

The shape of the ankle and foot should be inspected in the standing position. Movement should be observed in the sitting position since the range of ankle movement increases when the knee is bent.

The second metatarsal should point forward. The toes should be extended, i.e. flat on the floor and in line with their respective metatarsal bones. A longitudial arch should be visible on the medial side of the foot. The heel should be in line with the achilles tendon.

Figure 26. (A&B) Flexion/extension of the ankle.

The ankle is actively extended and then flexed. When maximal effort is used, the great toe usually extends and flexes as well.

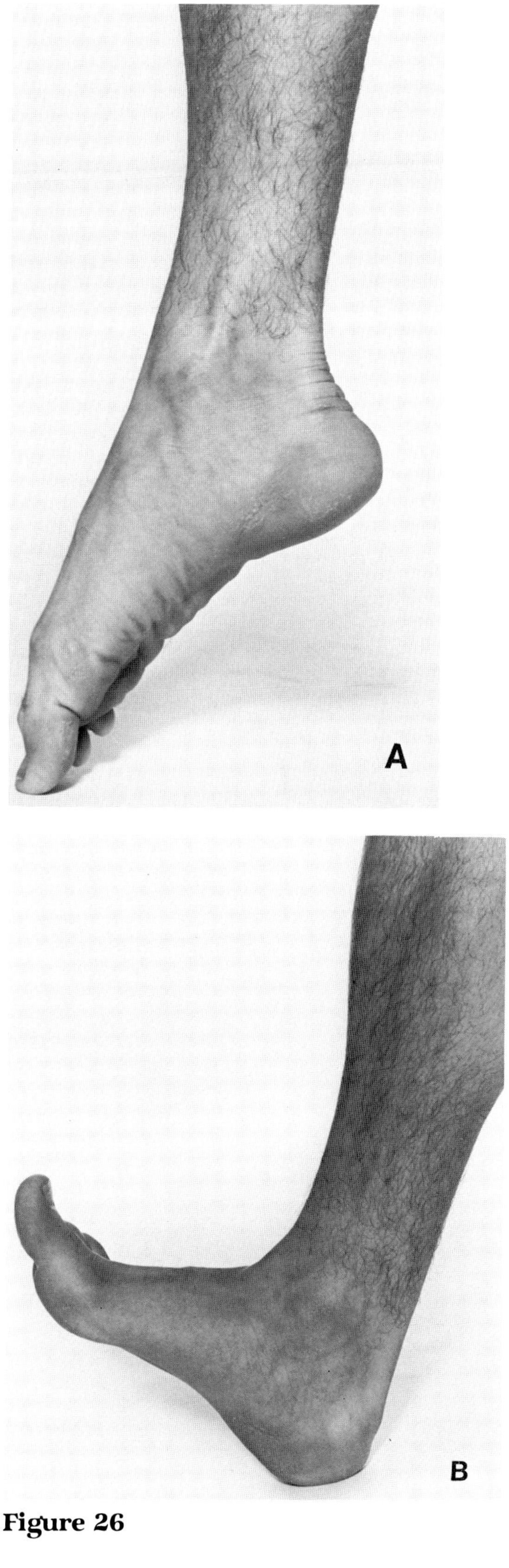

Figure 26

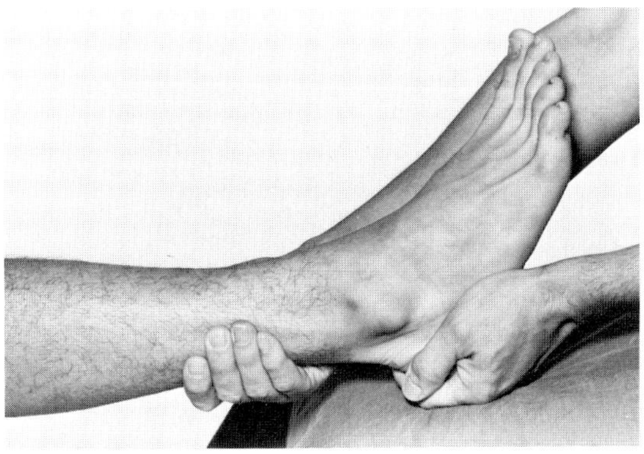

Figure 27

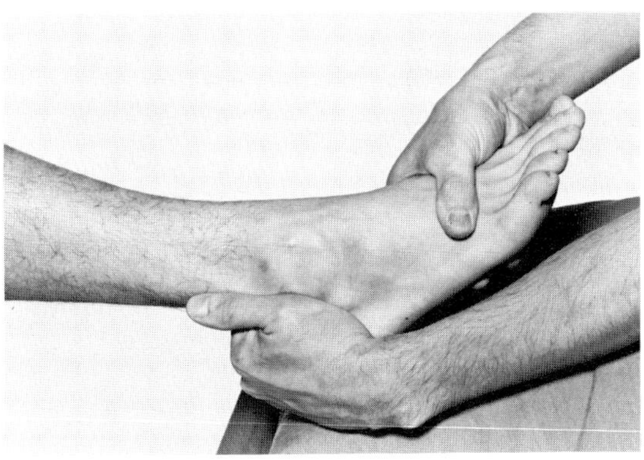

Figure 28

The Subtalar Joint

Figure 27. Passive movement of the subtalar joint.

The subtalar joint is best examined passively. The lower leg is supported with one hand while the other grasps the heel and moves it into eversion and inversion. The ankle should be in the neutral or slightly dorsiflexed position to prevent any coronal movement.

The Midtarsal Joint

Figure 28. Passive movement of the midtarsal joint.

The midtarsal joint is also examined passively. One hand holds the heel while the other grasps the forefoot at the level of the metatarsal necks and inverts and everts the forefoot on the hindfoot.

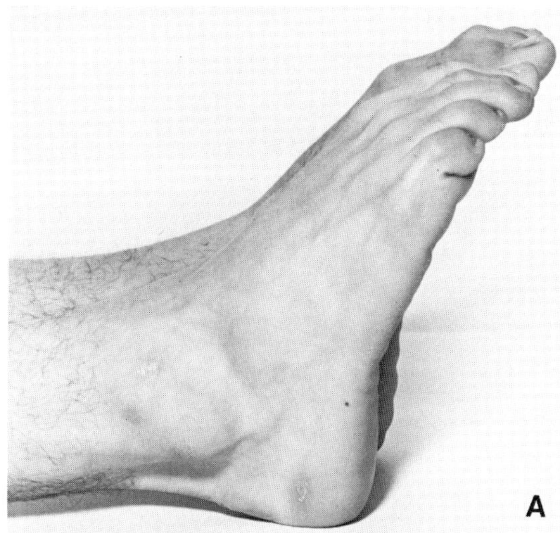

The Forefoot

Figure 29. (A&B) Flexion/extension of the toes.

The patient flexes and extends the toes to demonstrate mobility. The plantar surface is examined for callosities.

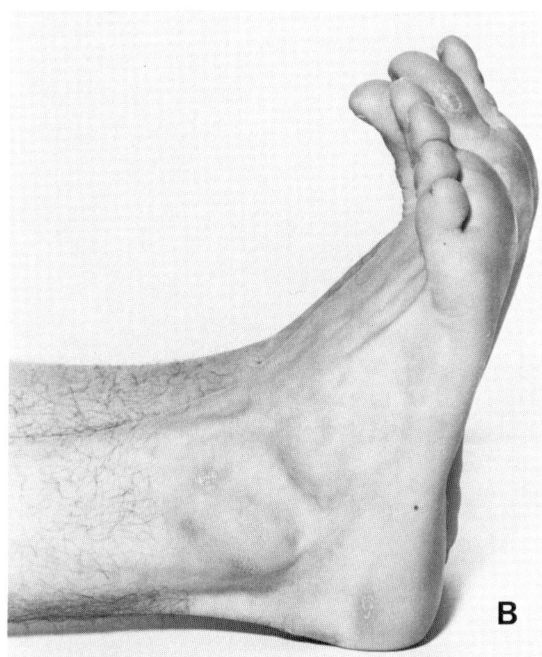

Figure 29

3

The Abnormal Joint

A joint at rest may show abnormalities of shape or size. During movement, a joint may show abnormalities of range of motion or kinetics. Inspection must be so structured that each of these abnormalities will be recognized. Palpation adds to the information obtained by inspection. Palpation includes active assisted and passive movements as well as diagnostic palpation. This chapter describes the visual and palpable findings in an abnormal joint.

INSPECTION AT REST

Abnormalities of Shape
- angulation
- translocation
- rotation
- length

Abnormalities of Size
- swelling localized
generalized
- atrophy localized
generalized

THE RHEUMATOLOGICAL PHYSICAL EXAMINATION
ISBN 0-8089-1824-9

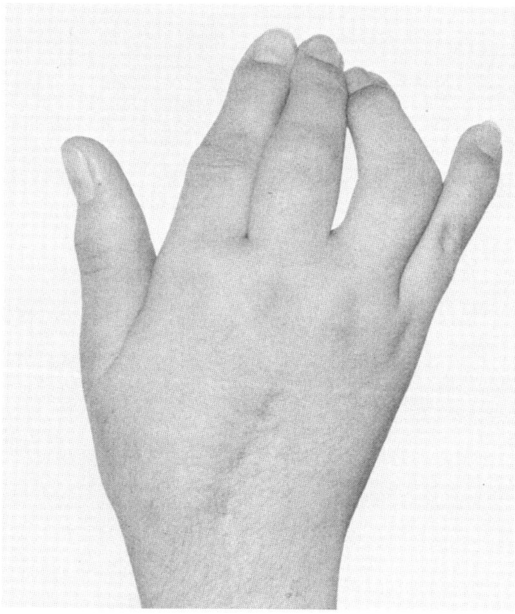

Figure 30

Abnormalities of Shape

Figure 30. Angulation of a P.I.P. joint.

Angulation is a deviation from normal alignment. In the extremities, the following terms have been used to describe angulation; valgus (deviation away from the midline), varus (deviation toward the midline), flexion deformity, extension deformity (recurvatum). Angulation of the spine is described with the following terms; lordosis (excessive extension), kyphosis (excessive flexion), scoliosis (deviation in the coronal plane, often S shaped).

Diagram 7. Planes and axes.

Angulation is described in reference to three body planes; the sagittal plane, the coronal plane and the horizontal plane. Rotation is described in reference to the longitudinal axis of the spine or the extremities.

7—Axes and Body Planes

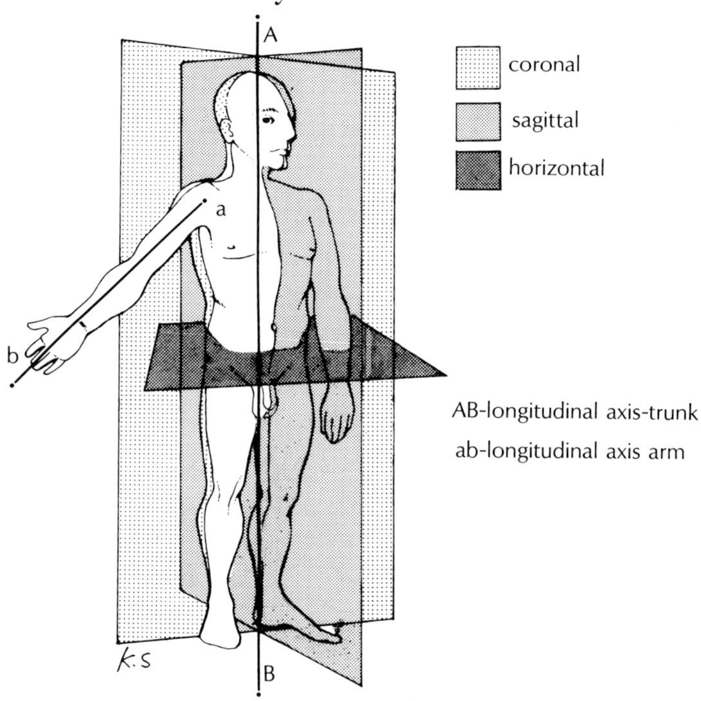

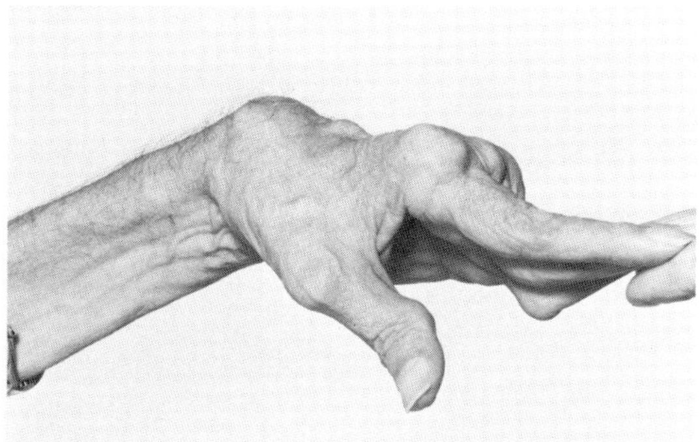

Figure 31

Figure 31. Translocation at wrist and M.C.P joints.

Translocation is the normal movement of a sliding joint. It becomes abnormal if it is excessive or if it occurs in an abnormal direction. Slight abnormalities are subluxations (partial luxation). When the normally opposing surfaces have slipped off one another completely it is a luxated or dislocated joint. Excessive translocation of one vertebra on another is called a spondylolisthesis.

Rotational deformities are often subtle. One needs a detailed knowledge of surface anatomy to determine the site of the rotatory abnormality. Rotational deformities of the extremities may arise from inadequate or excessive rotation during development. Rotational deformities of the spine are often associated with an angular deformity, the combined lesion is called a rotoscoliosis.

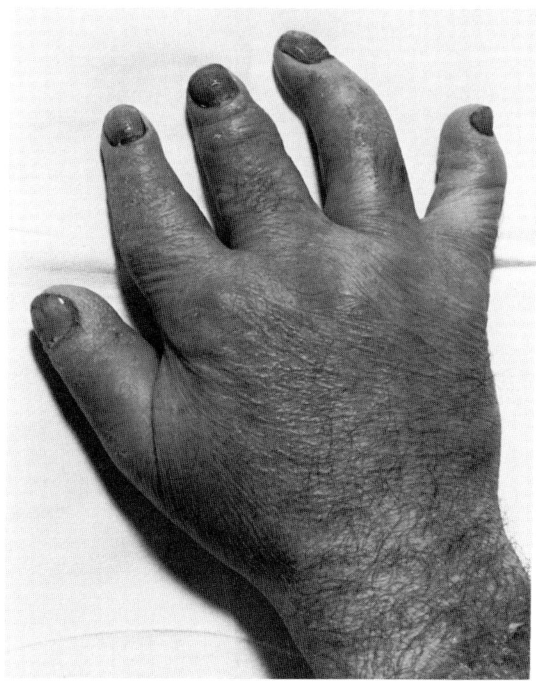

Figure 32

Figure 32. Loss of digital length.

Abnormalities of length may occur without malalignment. Developmental abnormalities may cause limbs that are short (e.g. achondroplasia) or long (e.g. Marfan's syndrome). Acquired shortening of the trunk or extremities is common and may be due to cartilage attrition or bone collapse or both. Acquired lengthening of a bone is rare.

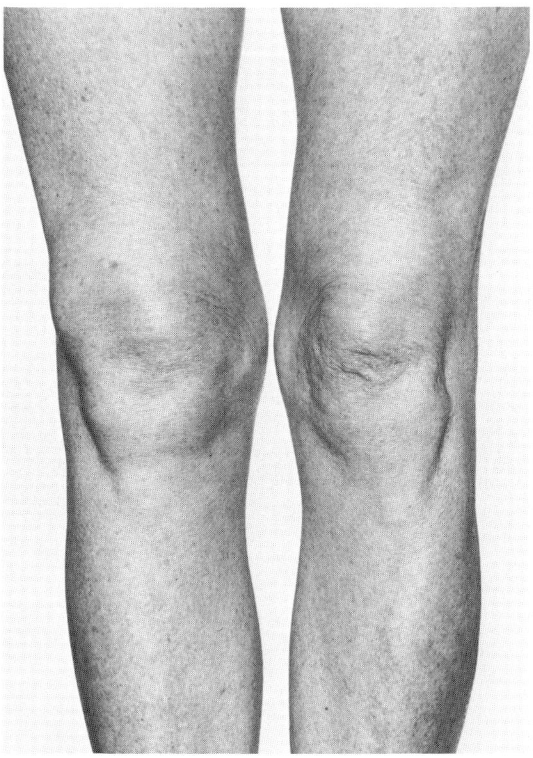

Figure 33

Abnormalities of Size

Figure 33. Intracapsular swelling of the knees.

Localized swelling is confined by an anatomical structure such as the joint capsule, a tendon sheath, or a bursa. Capsular distension can be seen in those joints that are close to the surface and one can appreciate that the capsule extends beyond the joint margins. Localized bony enlargement (osteophyte) may be intracapsular or extracapsular, often the enlargement is adjacent to the joint margin. The examiner must have a working knowledge of anatomy to recognize when a swelling is confined by the joint capsule.

Generalized swelling around joints is common and may have many causes. Injuries, infections, reflex dystrophies, acromegaly, and many other processes can cause generalized swelling, particularly in the dependent extremities.

The visible distribution of the swelling is seldom enough information for diagnosis. Observations made during movement and by palpation are usually required.

Atrophy around a joint is usually due to loss of muscle bulk, rarely it is due to atrophy of skin and subcutaneous tissue or faulty development. Mild regional atrophy of muscles commonly reflects disuse, marked localized muscle atrophy suggests denervation.

Scars and abnormal skin appendages or color should be noted.

4

The Temporomandibular Joint

Jack L. Stein

The temporomandibular joint is the only major diarthrodial joint between two membrane bones. It has three unique features;

1. Both articular surfaces are covered with fibrocartilage rather than hyaline cartilage
2. Condylar growth occurs in the deeper layers of this fibrocartilage without an epiphyseal plate such as that found in long bones
3. The joint is separated into two structural and functional compartments by a fibrocartilagenous disc

THE RHEUMATOLOGICAL PHYSICAL EXAMINATION
ISBN 0-8089-1824-9

10—The Mandible

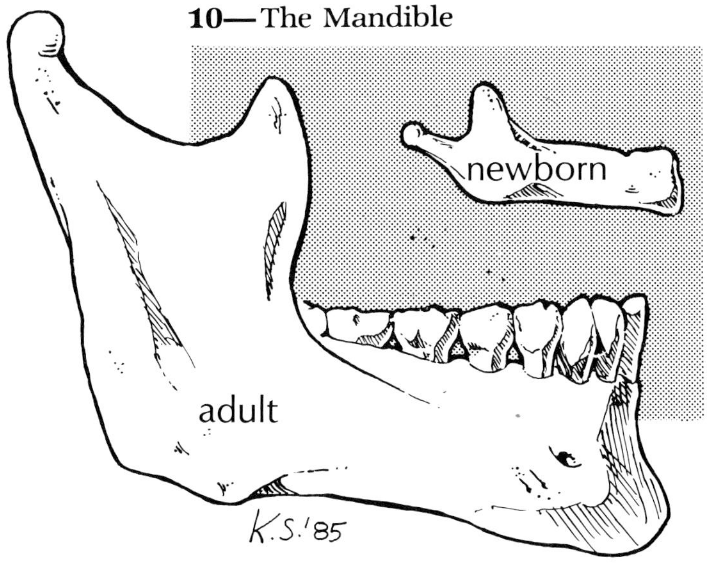

11—

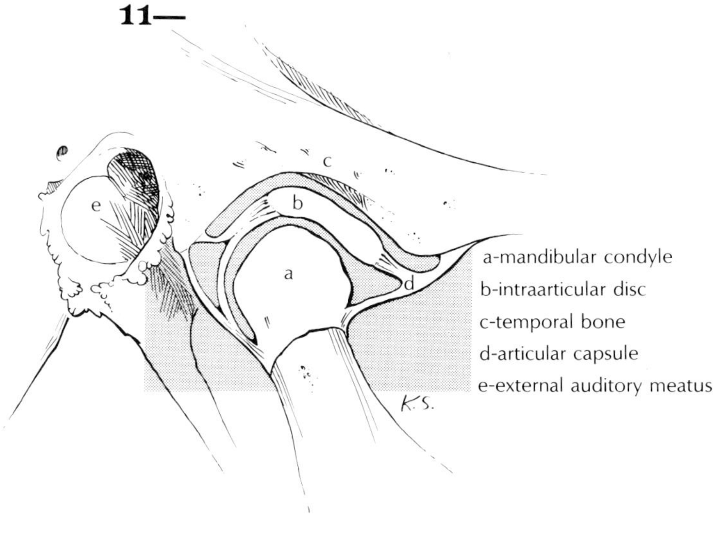

DEVELOPMENT AND DEVELOPMENTAL ABNORMALITIES

Diagram 10. The fetal and adult mandible.

Mesenchymal tissue condenses around Meckel's cartilage to form the body of the mandible and ossification begins at about the sixth week. By the 12th week, 2 cartilagenous ridges develop over the superior aspect of the mandible. These enlarge and ossify to form the condyle and the coronoid process. At birth, the two halves of the mandible are joined at the mental symphysis. There is continued growth at this symphysis for the first year and then the two halves fuse.

Growth and remodelling of the mandible continues into adult life. This seems to depend on the fibrocartilage over the condyle since injuries to this area result in faulty development of the whole hemi-mandible.

Hypoplasia (micrognathia) can be due to congenital agenesis (Pierre Robin Syndrome), to birth trauma to the growing condyle by forceps delivery, or to other mechanical or inflammatory processes. Unilateral hypoplasia causes facial asymmetry. A hypoplastic jaw opens inadequately and causes mal-occlusion.

Hyperplasia (prognathism) may be partial as in hemi-hypertrophy or complete as in pituitary gigantism or acromegaly.

FUNCTIONAL ANATOMY

Diagram 11. Anatomy of the temporomandibular joint.

Joint: The fibrocartilagenous disc allows the two compartments to function differently; the upper as a sliding joint, the lower as a hinge joint. On initial opening the condylar heads rotate, followed by forward sliding of the discs and condyles on the temporal articulations.

Ligaments: The capsule is reinforced by the strong lateral temporomandibular ligament that joins the neck of the mandible to the zygomatic process of the temporal bone. There are two weaker medial ligaments. The downward, backward course of the ligaments allows the condyle to swing down and forward.

Muscles: In the normal resting state, the jaw is held in place by the tonic contraction of the masticatory muscles and the teeth do not touch. The mouth is opened by contraction of the lateral pterygoid muscles with assistance from the submental strap muscles and gravity. The mouth is closed by the strong temporal, masseter, and medial pterygoid muscles. Selective use of these muscles allows the other movements of chewing. Normal chewing causes minimal pressure on the disc because of dental contact. However, a strong bite with the mouth wide open can compress the disc and cause severe pain. Excessively forced opening can dislocate the condyle anteriorly requiring passive relocation.

Diagram 12. Condylar position with the mouth open and closed.

12— Condylar Position

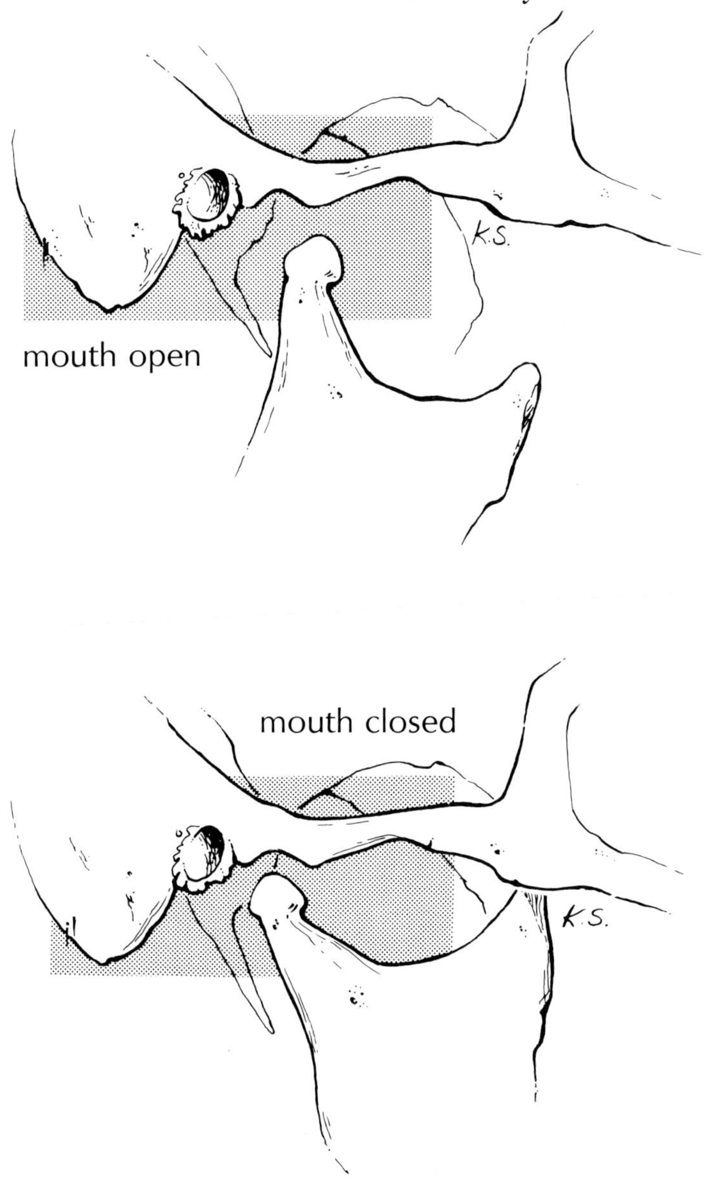

13—

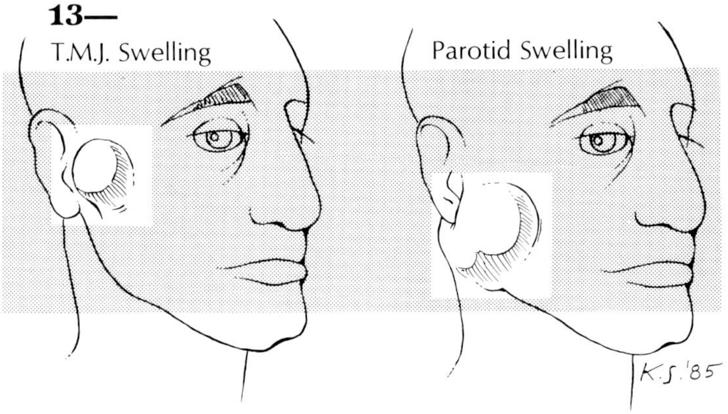

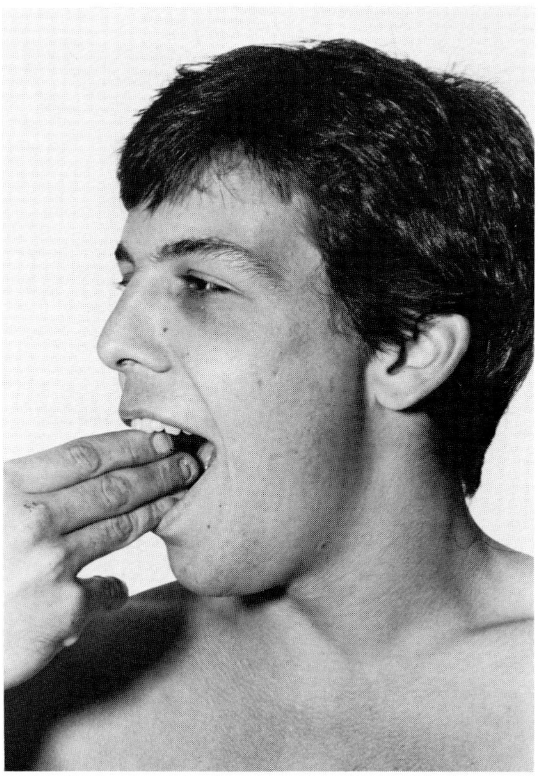

Figure 1

PHYSICAL EXAMINATION

Inspection at Rest

The jaw is observed to be symmetrical with the chin cleft in the midline. The cheek in front of the ear is flat when the mouth is closed. Swelling in the temporomandibular joint is localized just anterior to the tragus of the ear. Swelling of the parotid lies over the ramus of the mandible, extending backwards under the ear and forwards superficial to the masseter muscle. The whole cheek may be enlarged by simple obesity or the effect of excessive corticosteroids.

Diagram 13. Swelling of the temporomandibular joint.

The mouth should also be examined for abnormalities related to the temporomandibular joint. An absence of posterior teeth, unilaterally or bilaterally, may result in abnormal stresses on the temporomandibular joint during mastication.

Inspection with Movement

Figure 1. Demonstrates normal mouth opening.

In the adult the mouth normally opens to an interdental distance of 4–5 cms. When the mouth is opened, the condyle of the mandible forms a prominence in front of the ear. Slight asymmetry and slight interruption of movement are normal. Guarded, restricted opening suggests an inflamed joint. Guarded closing or biting suggests compression of the intra-articular disc or an unrelated dental problem.

Palpation

Active Assisted and Passive Movements

These are seldom required although they may help to determine whether restricted movement is due to muscle spasm.

Diagnostic Palpation

Two fingers are placed on the posterior part of the zygomatic arch and moved posteriorly. The bony arch slants inwardly and the fingers press against the cartilage of the tragus of the ear. The mandibular condyle is felt as a firm swelling below and behind the inward slant of the arch. Moving caudally, one can feel the upper part of the ramus of the mandible running almost perpendicular to the zygomatic arch,

As the mouth is opened one can feel the round condyle moving down and forward leaving a slight hollow (finger tip size) between the ear and the condyle.

The posterior aspect of the temporomandibular joint is examined by placing the tip of the little finger into the external auditory canal. Palpating anteriorly, one can feel the condyle moving as the mouth opens and closes.

The joint capsule is palpated for distension, tenderness and heat. If there is an effusion, the normal hollow may not develop as the mouth is opened. The bony margins of the condyle and the temporal bone are palpated for enlargement. Spasm and/or hypertrophy of the temporal and masseter muscles may be detected.

Crepitus

Many people feel painless crepitus or hear an audible snap as the condyles slide forward under the temporal eminence. Painful crepitus suggests that the disc is being compressed or that the disc and cartilage are eroded allowing the condyle and the temporal bone to come into contact.

5

The Neck and Back

Hugh Little

DEVELOPMENT

Prenatal

The axial skeleton develops before the extremities. At 3 weeks the notocord forms a rod like structure in the middle of the embryonic disc with plates of mesoderm on each side. These plates segment to form primitive vertebrae with the medial part surrounding the notocord and then extending dorsally and laterally around the neural canal to form the arch and costal processes.

The mesenchymal cells in the upper spinal segments begin to form cartilage at about the 7th week. Soon after, ossification begins. Each cartilagenous ring has 3 ossification centres, one anteriorly corresponding to the vertebral body and one on each side in the pedicle area of the neural arch (see Chapter 1). The atlas has two lateral ossification centres. The odontoid has paired ossification centres that coalesce and fuse with the axis during the third or forth year.

THE RHEUMATOLOGICAL PHYSICAL EXAMINATION
ISBN 0-8089-1824-9

The costal process of the vertebra is rudimentary in the cervical and lumbar area where it is incorporated in the transverse process. In the thorax, the costal processes elongate to form the ribs and in the sacrum they form the massive lateral part of the fused vertebrae.

14—Vertebral Growth Plates

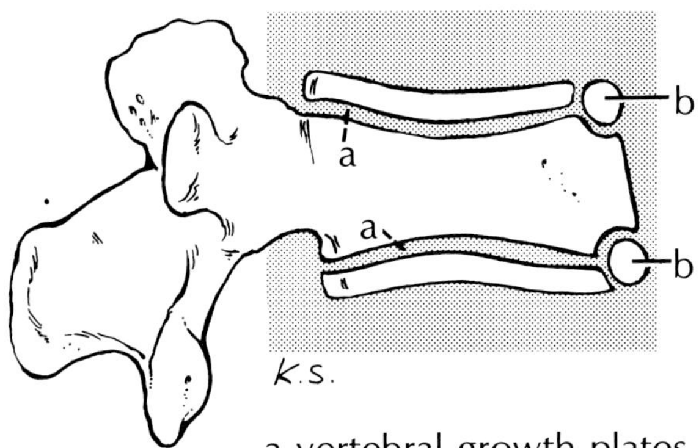

a-vertebral growth plates
b-ring apophysis

Postnatal Development

At birth the vertebrae are shaped alike. The regional differences develop as they grow.

At about a year, the lateral ossification centres fuse posteriorly to form the bony neural arch. Growth continues in the neurocentral joints until the fifth year enlarging the arch.

Diagram 14. Vertebral growth plates.

Longitudinal growth of the vertebral bodies continues at the growth plates near the cephalic and caudal ends of each vertebra. At age 10 another ossification centre (ring apophysis) develops around the edges of the vertebral bodies and fuses at about age 18. Circumferential growth of the vertebra through subperiosteal apposition is similar to other long bones.

DEVELOPMENTAL ABNORMALITIES

Segmentation failure	total	block vertebrae Klippel-Feil
	partial	angulation and rotational deformities
Neural Arch failure	meningomyelocoele spinal stenosis Epiphyseal failure Morquio's Syndrome spondyloepiphyseal dysplasia	
Duplication	diastomatomyelia	

FUNCTIONAL ANATOMY

Vertebrae

The vertebrae protect the spinal cord and the viscera and allow movement of the neck and back.

The vertebrae from C3 to L5 have a common pattern. They have an anterior vertebral body, a posterior neural arch that has transverse processes laterally and a single spinous process posteriorly. The neural arch has facet joints above and below.

Diagram 15. Cervical, thoracic, and lumbar vertebrae seen from above.

The cervical vertebrae can be recognized by the foramen for the vertebral arteries in the transverse processes. C3 to C7 have a bony ridge on the suprolateral margin of the vertebral body for the uncovertebral joints (of Luschka).

The thoracic vertebrae can be recognized by the long transverse processes that are directed posteriorly and have articular facets near the tip for the ribs. The thoracic vertebral bodies are somewhat wedge shaped and have articular facets on the posterior corners for the base of the ribs.

The lumbar vertebral bodies are kidney shaped. The facet joints are oriented in the sagittal plane and the spinous process is thick, short and points straight back.

Diagram 16. The atlas and axis.

The atlas (C1) and axis (C2) differ from the usual pattern. The atlas is a ring that encloses two longitudinal structures; the spinal cord posteriorly and the odontoid process of the axis anteriorly. The lateral masses of the atlas are wedge shaped thickenings that support the articular surfaces of the occipital condyles above and the axis below. The axis differs from the usual pattern by virtue of the odontoid process projecting cranially from the superior surface of the vertebral body.

15—Vertebrae, Seen from Above

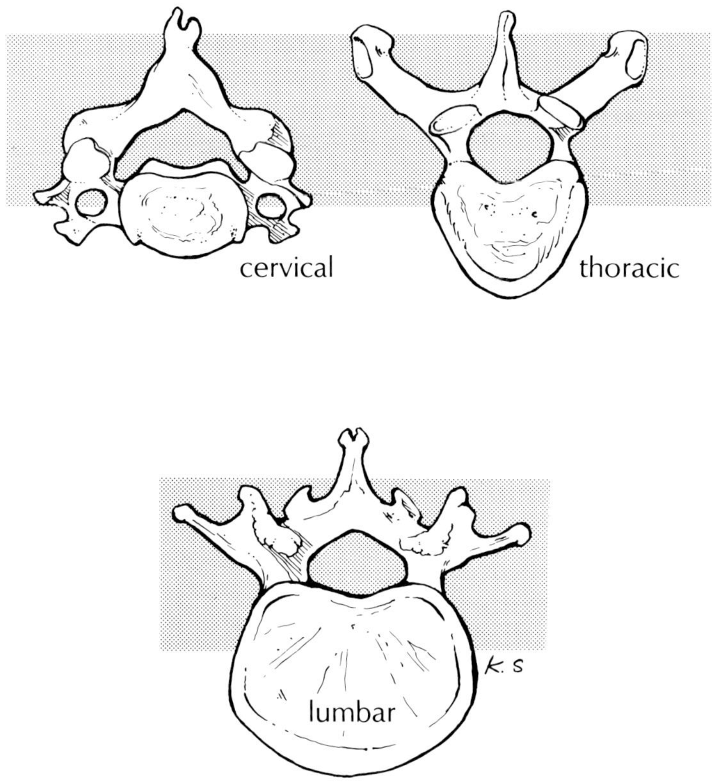

16—Atlas and Axis

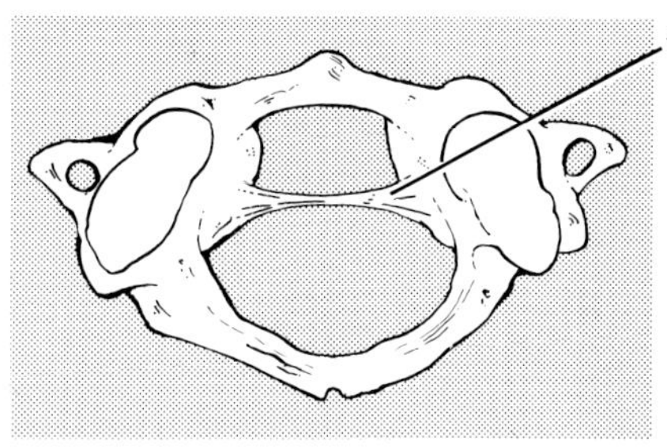

Atlas, superior aspect

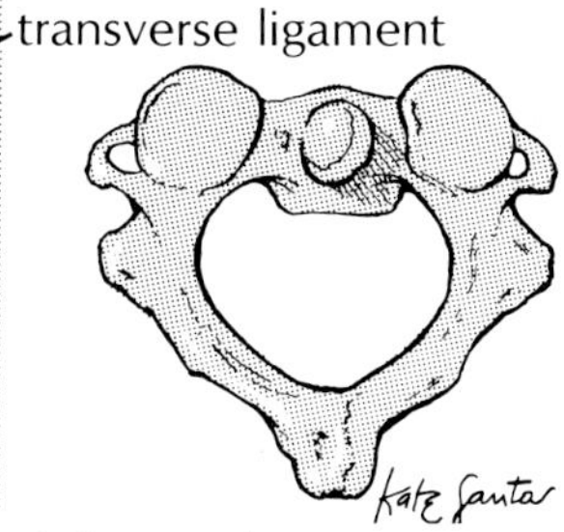
Axis, superior aspect

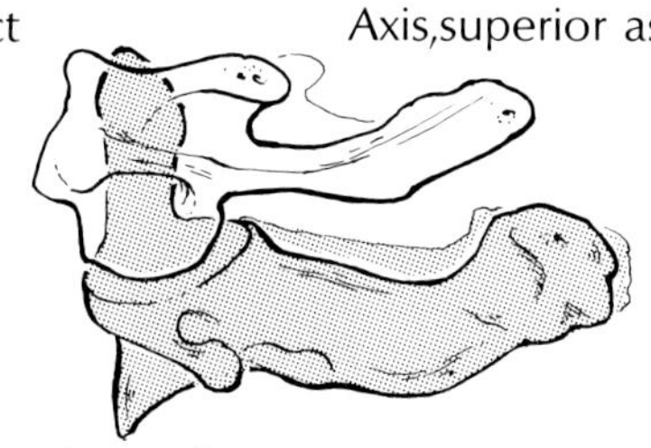
atlas and axis;
lateral view, showing the odontoid process

17— Intervertebral Ligaments

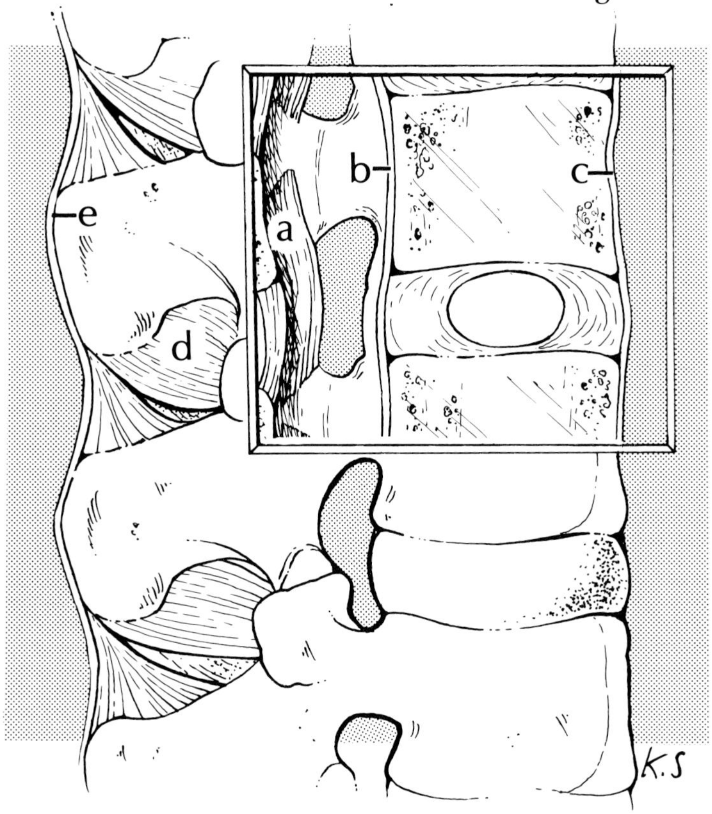

a - ligamentum flavum
b - posterior longitudinal ligament
c - anterior longitudinal ligament
d - interspinous ligament
e - supraspinous ligament

Joints

The intervertebral discs are complex symphyses. The facets and uncovertebral joints are sliding joints that limit the movement at that segment.

Diagram 17. The intervertebral ligaments.

Ligaments

The spine is reinforced by numerous ligaments. The anterior and posterior longitudinal ligaments run the length of the spine from the basi-occiput to the sacrum attaching to each vertebral body and each disc. The neural arches are connected by segmental ligaments. The lamina are connected by the ligamentum flavum, the transverse processes by the intertransverse ligament, the facets by the joint capsule, the spinous process by the inter and supraspinous ligaments. There are ligamentous reinforcements at both the costovertebral joints and the spino-pelvic junction.

Muscles

The spine is surrounded by several layers of longitudinal muscles joining adjacent segments and spanning several segments. The extensor muscles are particularly numerous and strong. The supra and infra hyoid muscles assist in flexion of the neck by pulling the chin toward the sternum. Thoracic flexion is assisted by the pectoralis minor and the lower fibres of the pectoralis major, both of which pull the shoulder girdle downward and forward. The muscles of the abdominal wall are the main lumbar flexors, assisted by the iliopsoas when the hips and pelvis are stabilized. Rotation is produced by the truncal and limb girdle muscles. Muscles that rotate the head and C1 on the neck join the large transverse processes of C1 to the occiput and the spinous process of C2.

MOVEMENTS

The spine can flex and extend in the sagittal plane and laterally flex in the coronal plane. It can rotate around the longitudinal axis and can increase or decrease its length by flattening or accentuating the spinal curves.

The cranio-cervical junction is distinctive. The rounded occipital condyles move on the cupped superior surface of the atlas to produce a discrete nodding movement of about 30 degrees. The atlantoaxial joint allows a discrete rotatory movement of the head and C1 on the neck of about 30 degrees.

Movement of the spine below the cranio-cervical junction involves distortion of the discs and sliding movement of the facet joints. The structure of the vertebrae facilitate certain movements at different levels. Sagittal flexion-extension is concentrated in the lower cervical and lower lumbar segments at the apices of the lordotic curves. Lateral flexion is greatest in the neck and rotation is greatest in the lower thoracic area.

PHYSICAL EXAMINATION OF THE NECK AND BACK

Stance and posture relate to the whole spine and are described in Chapter 16. The examination of the functional units; the neck, the thoracic spine and the lumbar spine, will be described in this chapter.

The Neck

The neck is examined from the front, back and side. Only the lower cervical spinous processes are visible so that the examination is limited to the relationship of the head to the trunk.

Angulation in a forward or lateral direction is common. The adolescent slouch, the senile kyphosis, the flexed spine of a spondylitic all angle the lower cervical spine forward and cause a compensatory hyperextension at the cranio-cervical junction. If marked, this may result in visible prominence of the posterior cervical muscles and horizontal soft tissue folds below the occiput.

Lateral angulation may be associated with rotation. The sternomastoid muscle should be inspected since a contracture will produce this deformity.

The neck may appear long if the trapezius is relaxed and the spinal curves are flat. The neck may appear short due to accentuated curves and elevation of the shoulder girdle. Developmental abnormalities may cause a short neck.

Inspection with Movement

Figures 3&4. Neck movements.

Loss of lateral flexion and rotation of the neck is common in the elderly due to degeneration of the discs, the unco-vertebral joints, and the facet joints. This loss is accentuated if the neck is in the extended position and the facet joints are closely packed.

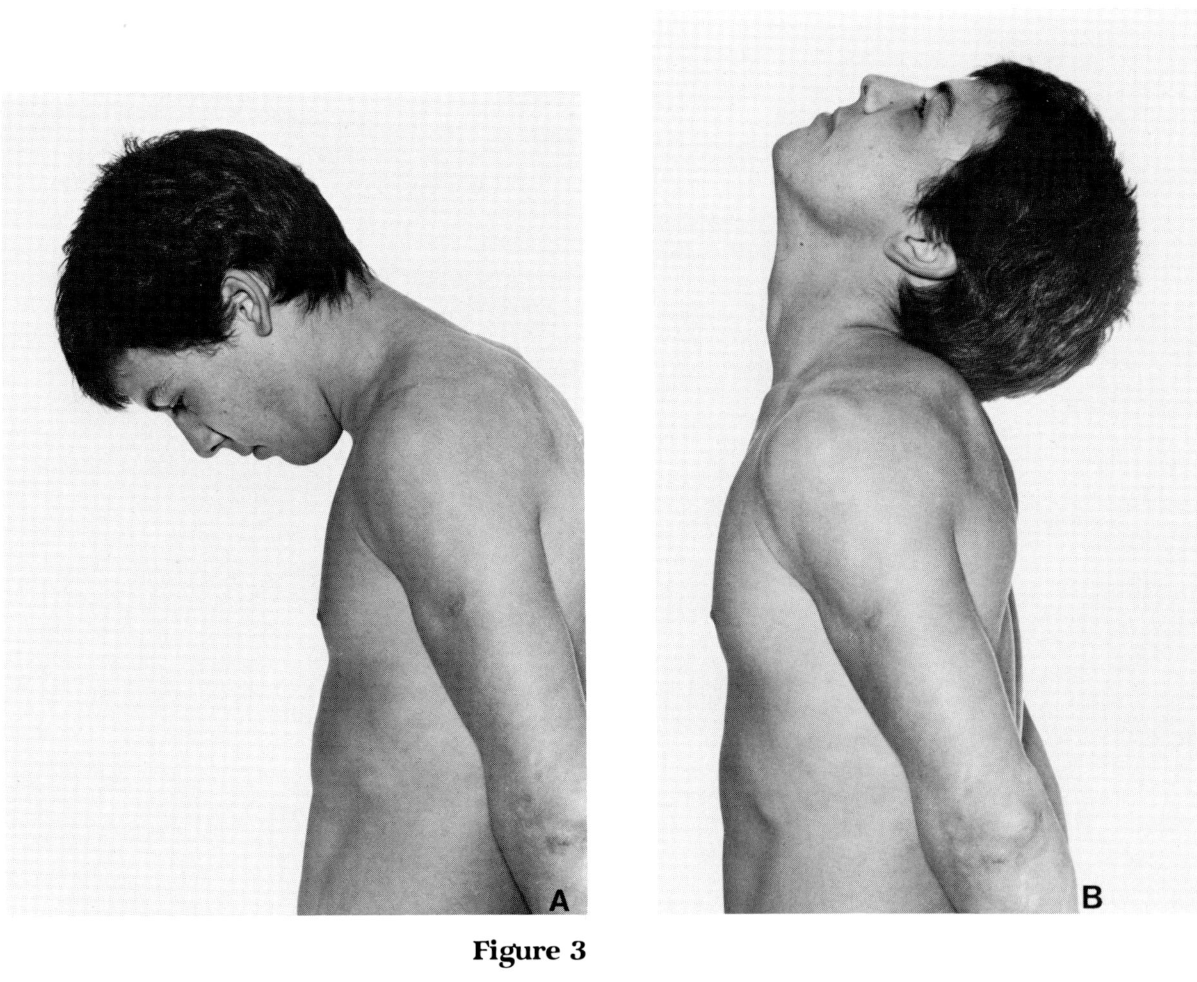

Figure 3

Chest Expansion

The ribs move on the spine and the sternum. Reduced chest cage movement is usually the result of intrathoracic events but joint disease can cause restriction.

A circumferential measurement should be made at the level of the 4th intercostal space anteriorly. The measurement is made in both full inspiration and full expiration and the difference is recorded. The patient stands with the hands resting on or behind the head. Expansion of 4 cms., or more is normal in an adult male.

Figure 34. Measurement of chest expansion (A) expiration; (B) inspiration.

The Lumbar Spine

Inspection at Rest

The lumbar spine should be inspected from the side and the back. The vertebral spinous processes are seldom visible but their position can be deduced by the groove between the prominent paraspinal muscles. Angulations are noted relative to the occipital axis. Rotational deformities are usually combined with some angulation.

Inspection with Movement

The lumbar spine provides most of the sagittal flexion/extension of the trunk. In the fully flexed position the lumbar spine forms a smooth curve from the sacrum to the thorax. Tight hamstrings prevent full flexion of the hips and also appear to limit lumbar flexion as well. If flexion is limited, slight bending of the knees can increase range.

Note the kinetics of flexion and extension. Patients with vertebral body compression fractures resist flexion. Patients with facet impingement pain complain as they initiate extension from the fully flexed position and complain again on hyperextension in the erect position.

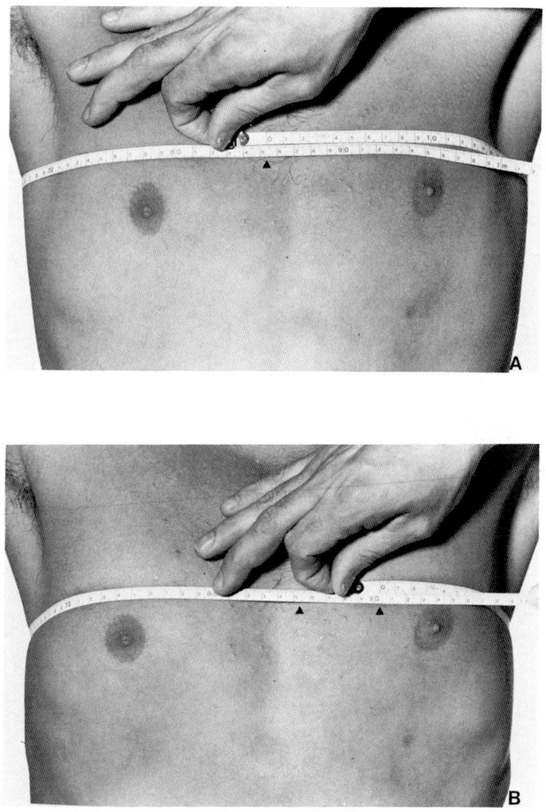

Figure 34

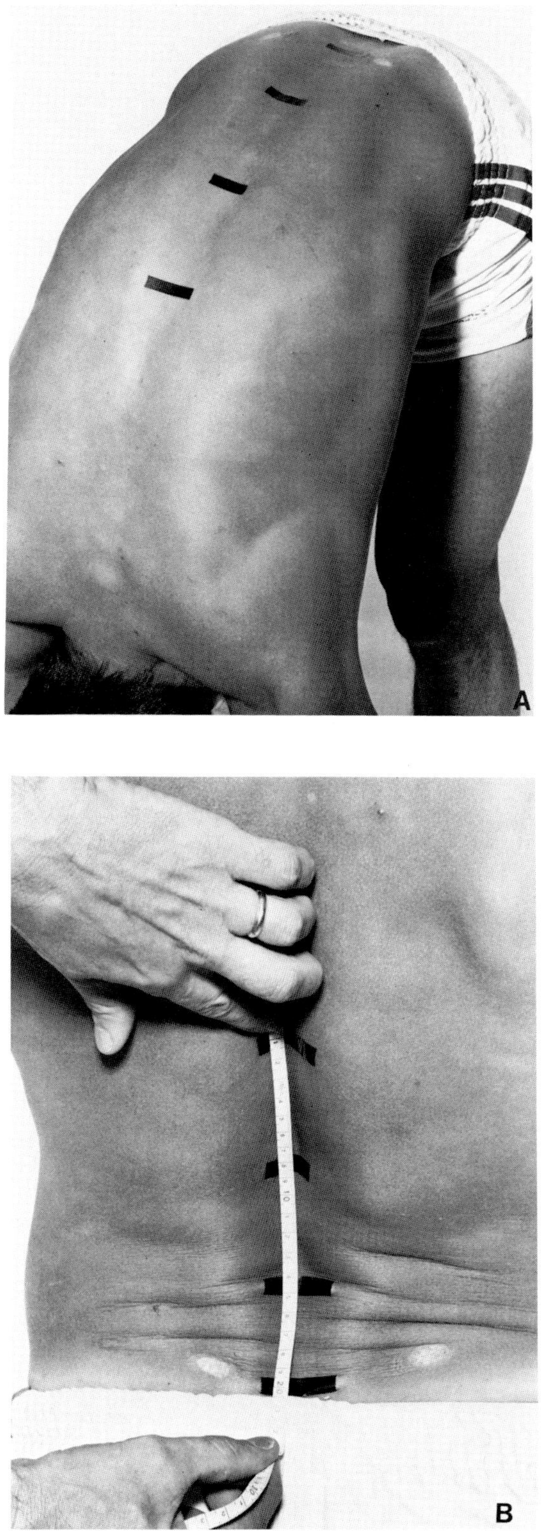

Figure 35

Diagnostic Palpation

Abnormalities of shape are measured. Lateral flexion is measured as the distance from the middle finger tip to the upper edge of the fibula with the patient in maximal lateral flexion (finger–fibula test). The patient must not bend forward and both heels must stay on the floor.

Flexion/extension of the lumbar spine is measured by the modified Shober test.

Figure 35. (A&B) The modified Shober test.

The patient flexes foreward as far as possible. Starting at an upper sacral spinous prominence, three 10 cm. segments are measured and marked on the spine. The patient stands erect and the distance between the marks is measured again. The lowest segment should shorten by at least 50%. The middle and upper segments shorten by 40 and 30% respectively. The amount of shortening is greater in tall individuals.

If this movement is restricted in the erect position it should be repeated with flexion measured in the sitting position and extension in the prone 'push-up' position. This may lessen pain, allowing a greater range of motion.

Diagram 24. The Shober test in the sitting/prone position (after Smythe).

Loss of height can be assessed by, noting the relationship of the costal margin to the iliac crest in the mid axillary line. There is normally a space of 3 to 5 cms. Minor loss is difficult to assess but a significant loss will obliterate this space causing the rib cage to rest on the inside of the iliac crest

With the patient in the prone slightly flexed position, translocations may be palpable as a step in the normal smooth alignment of the spinous processes. Deep pressure over the spinous processes and the interspinous ligaments can cause pain, localizing areas of damage. Palpation for tenderness should include the soft tissue in the costovertebral angle and the tissues over the posterior iliac spines.

A complete examination of the spine includes a rectal examination to examine the coccyx, manipulate the sacrococcygeal joint as well as to assess the tone and power of the rectal sphincter for weakness, suggesting sacral nerve dysfunction.

Spinal disease may affect the spinal cord or the spinal nerve roots. The symptoms and signs of spinal cord lesions, nerve root irritation and nerve root dysfunction are described in the references in the Reading List.

24—Modified Shober Test, Sitting-Prone Position (after Smythe)

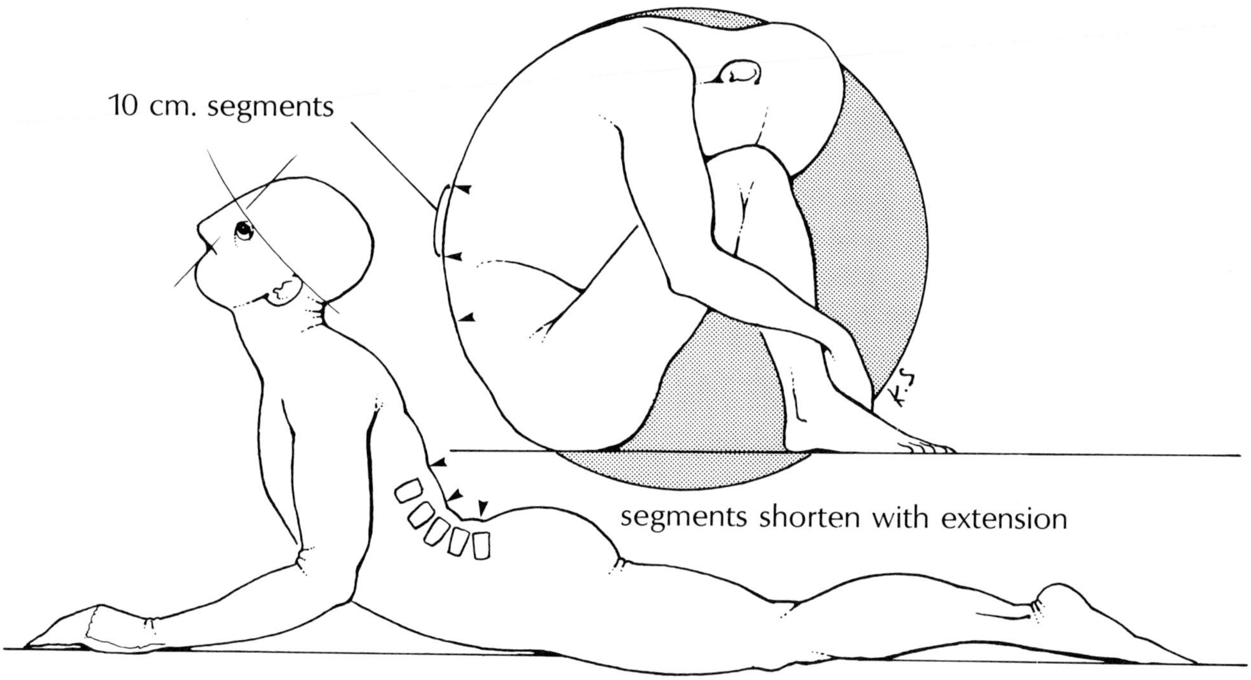

6

The Shoulder Girdle

Joseph B. Houpt

DEVELOPMENT OF THE SHOULDER GIRDLE

The upper limb bud appears during the 4th week of embryonic development. From an initial cervical position, the scapula descends down over the ribs and arrives at its final location at about the 12th week. Congenital abnormalities occur from failure of development or migration of the components of the limb bud.

DEVELOPMENTAL ABNORMALITIES

Anomalies of the Scapula

1. Sprengel's Deformity—The scapula rides at an abnormally high level, often with a bony or ligamentous connection to the spine because of failure of the normal descent of the limb bud.
2. Bipartite Acromion
3. Aplasia of the Glenoid

THE RHEUMATOLOGICAL PHYSICAL EXAMINATION
ISBN 0-8089-1824-9

25—The Shoulder Girdle, Superior Aspect

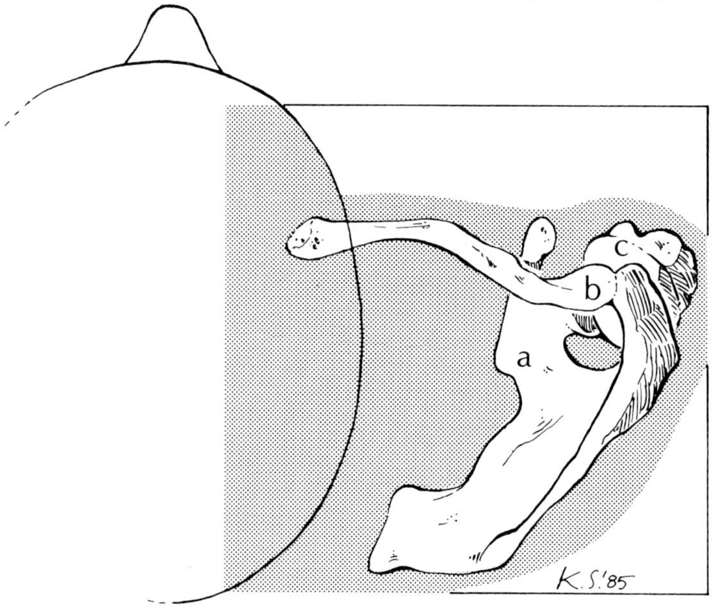

Anomalies of the Clavicle

1. Congenital coracoclavicular bar—A bar of bone develops and persists between the clavicle and the coracoid process.
2. Congenital pseudarthrosis of the Clavicle—a gap may persist between the two ossification centers at the junction of the outer 1/3 and the inner 2/3 of the clavicle.
3. Cleidocranial Dysostosis—Ineffective ossification of the clavicles and the skull leads to a varying degree of aplasia of the clavicles. The clavicles may be entirely absent making it possible to swing the two shoulders forward so that the arms touch anteriorly. Only the central part of the clavicle may be absent, appearing as a central pseudarthrosis.
4. Subluxation of the acromioclavicular joint.

FUNCTIONAL ANATOMY

Diagram 25. The shoulder girdle

Posterior Aspect

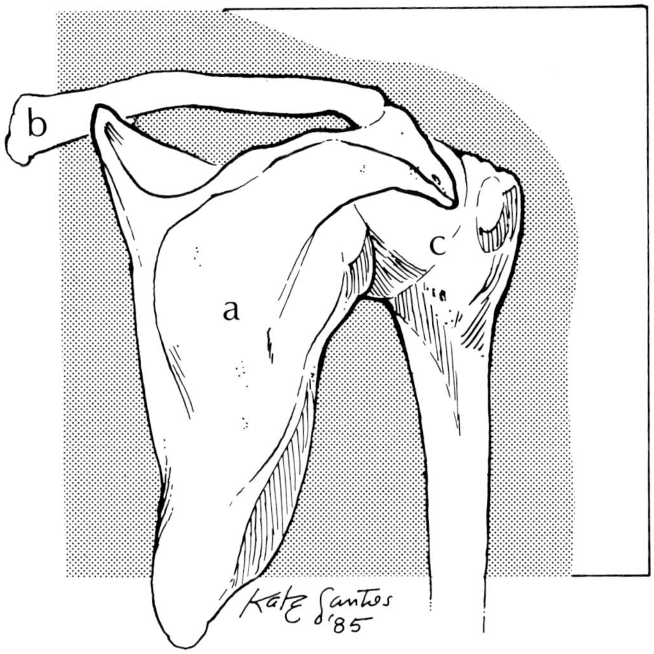

Bones

The bones of the shoulder girdle are the scapula (with its acromion and coracoid processes) and the clavicle. These bones articulate with the axial skeleton through the sternum and ribs.

The scapula (shoulder blade) is shaped like an axe head with the blade directed posteromedially. The lateral surface has a small, slightly concave articular surface for the head of the humerus. This glenoid fossa is deepened by a rim of cartilage, the glenoid labrum.

The scapula has two bony projections; the spine projects posteriorly and laterally ending in the acromion that angles forward like a beckoning finger, the coracoid process arises from the superior border and resembles a finger pointing directly forward. The spine of the scapula can be palpated throughout its length. The tip of the coracoid can be located just below the outer end of the clavicle.

The clavicle is an S-shaped bone with flattened curves. It acts as a strut, anchoring the scapula in its lateral position. There are articulations at both ends.

Anterior Aspect

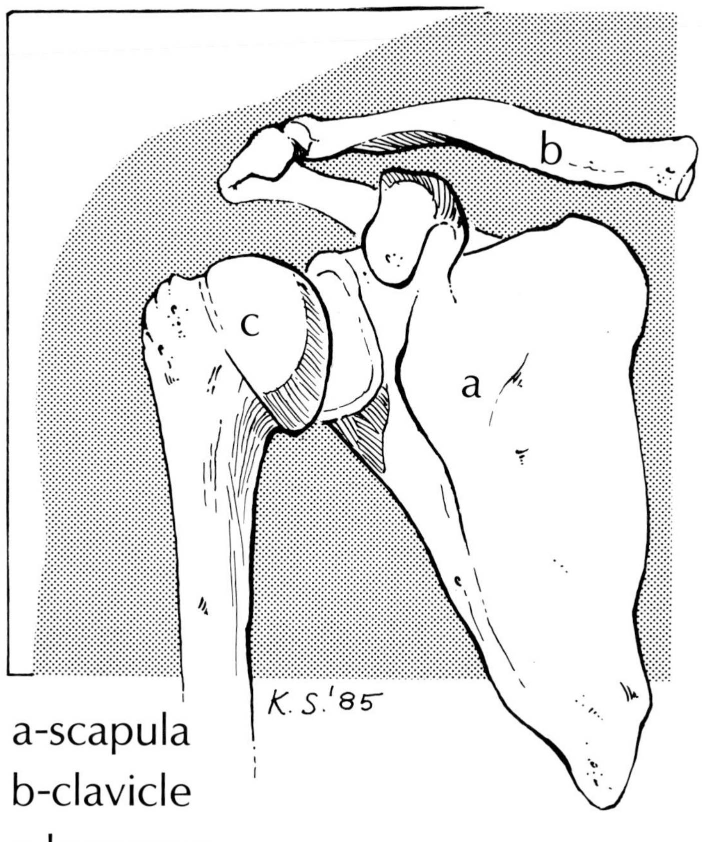

a-scapula
b-clavicle
c-humerus

26—The Acromioclavicular Joint

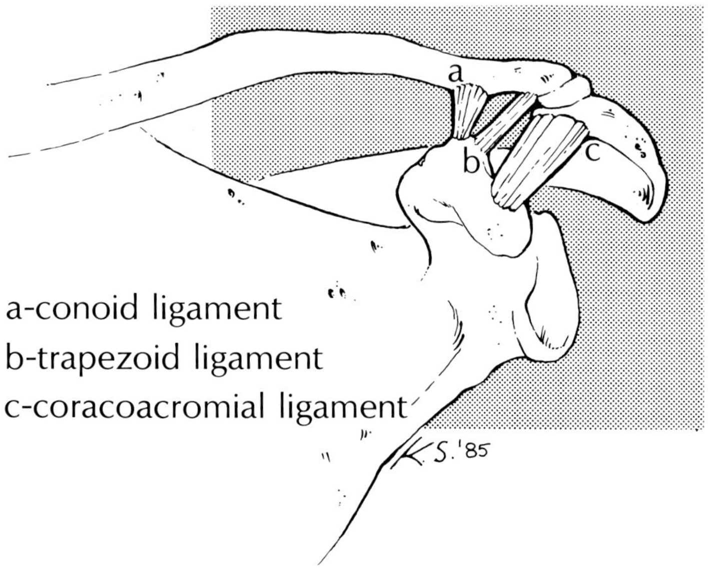

27—The Sternoclavicular Joint

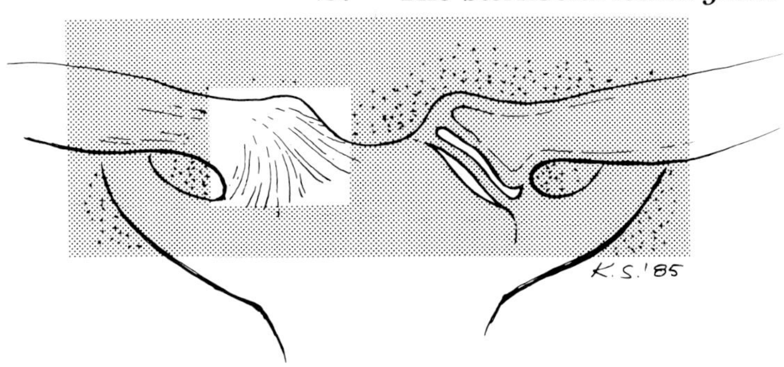

Joints

Diagram 26. The acromioclavicular joint.

The acromioclavicular joint has a small flat articular surface that is usually angled so that the clavicle tends to slide over the acromion. A fibrocartilagenous ring resembling an intra-articular meniscus develops over the first two decades. The disc and the articular surfaces undergo degenerative changes by the fourth decade.

Diagram 27. The sternoclavicular joint.

The sternum has a saddle shaped articular surface, enlarged by an intra-articular fibrocartilagenous disc to accomodate the articular surface on the medial end of the clavicle.

Ligaments

The clavicle is firmly attached to the scapula by the two parts of the coracoclavicular ligament. The lateral "trapezoid" and the medial "conoid" join the coracoid to the undersurface of the distal clavicle. They limit scapular rotation around the acromioclavicular joint and maintain a constant relationship of the scapula to the clavicle.

Sternoclavicular stability depends on the costoclavicular ligament that attaches the undersurface of the medial clavicle to the first rib. This ligament prevents the clavicle from slipping up and in, over the suprasternal notch.

Muscles

The scapula is suspended in a muscular sling and moves in a gliding fashion on the posterior ribcage. The upper, middle, and lower parts of the trapezius raise, retract, and lower the scapula respectively. The serratus anterior pulls the angle of the scapula forward and the rhomboids and levator scapulae pull it back. The pectoralis minor pulls the coracoid downward and forward depressing the shoulder girdle and rotating the scapula.

28—Surface Anatomy of the Shoulder Girdle

Anterior Aspect

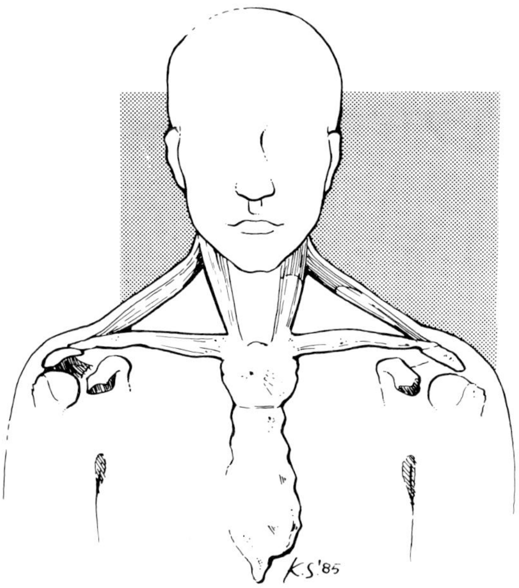

Both ends of the clavicle are obscured by muscles; the trapezius laterally and the sternocleidomastoid medially.

Posterior Aspect

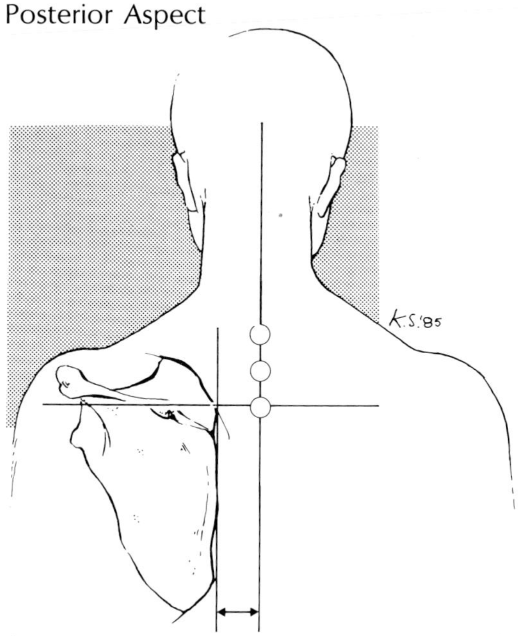

The spine of the scapula is at the level of the third thoracic spinous process. The medial border of the scapula is parallel to the spine, about 5 cms. lateral. With abduction of the shoulder, the angle of the scapula swings laterally.

MOVEMENTS

The clavicular joints allow both hinging and rotatory movements. Flexion of the sternoclavicular joint in the coronal plane (shoulder shrug) results in the opposite movement at the acromioclavicular joint. Elevation of the arm rotates the scapula and the clavicle due to its attachment through the coracoclavicular ligaments. The first 30 degrees of clavicular elevation occurs as flexion at the sternoclavicular joint. The next 30 degrees of elevation occurs by rotation of the clavicle along its long axis.

PHYSICAL EXAMINATION

Inspection at Rest

Diagram 28. Surface anatomy of the shoulder girdle.

Observe the patient from the back and the front. Identify the scapulae and note whether the medial borders are parallel to the spine and equi-distant from the spine. Are the medial borders applied to the chest wall or are they protruding? Draw an imaginary line joining the spinous processes of the scapulae. Is it horizontal? Does it cross the spine a few cms., below the vertebra prominens? If the scapulae are not symmetrically applied to the back, look for a scoliosis.

From the front one can identify the whole superior surface of the clavicle. The enlarged medial ends form the margins of the suprasternal notch. The acromioclavicular joint is usually inconspicuous but there may be a visible step down from the clavicle to the acromion without a subluxation.

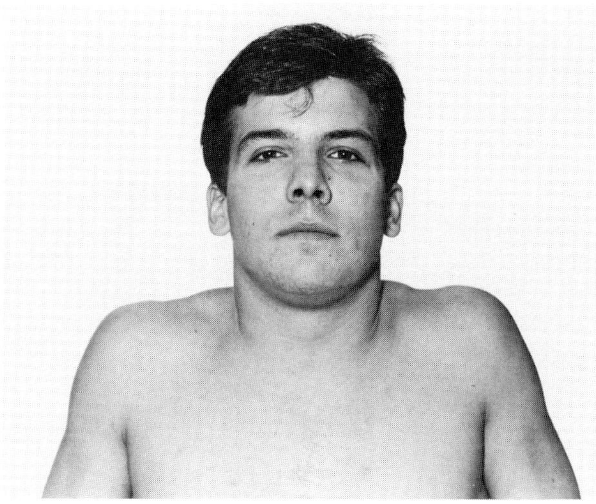

Figure 5

Inspection with Movement

Figure 5. The shoulder shrug.

The shoulder shrug tests mobility of the scapula on the thorax. Shoulder girdle movement amplifies the range of movement possible at the shoulder joint.

Palpation

The clavicle is palpated throughout its length. The joints are palpated for abnormalities of size, tenderness or crepitus. Instability of the sternoclavicular joint can be felt as a medial migration of the clavicle over the sternum as the shoulder girdle is protruded. Instability of the acromioclavicular joint can be felt as a lateral migration of the clavicle over the acromion when the arm is elevated.

The scapula should be palpated during movement of the shoulder girdle. If movement is restricted, the upper medial border should be carefully examined for a fibrous or bony attachment to the spine. The scapula is elevated in this uncommon condition.

7

The Shoulder

Joseph B. Houpt

DEVELOPMENT

As man climbed the evolutionary ladder, significant changes occured in the humerus. The upper end rotated so that the articular surface faces medially rather than dorsally. The distal humerus rotated externally so that the humeral epicondyles approach the coronal plane.

Ossification begins in the humeral head during the 1st year, the greater tuberosity during the 3rd year and the lesser tuberosity during the 5th year. The epiphysis fuses at age 20.

THE RHEUMATOLOGICAL PHYSICAL EXAMINATION
ISBN 0-8089-1824-9

29—The Shoulder

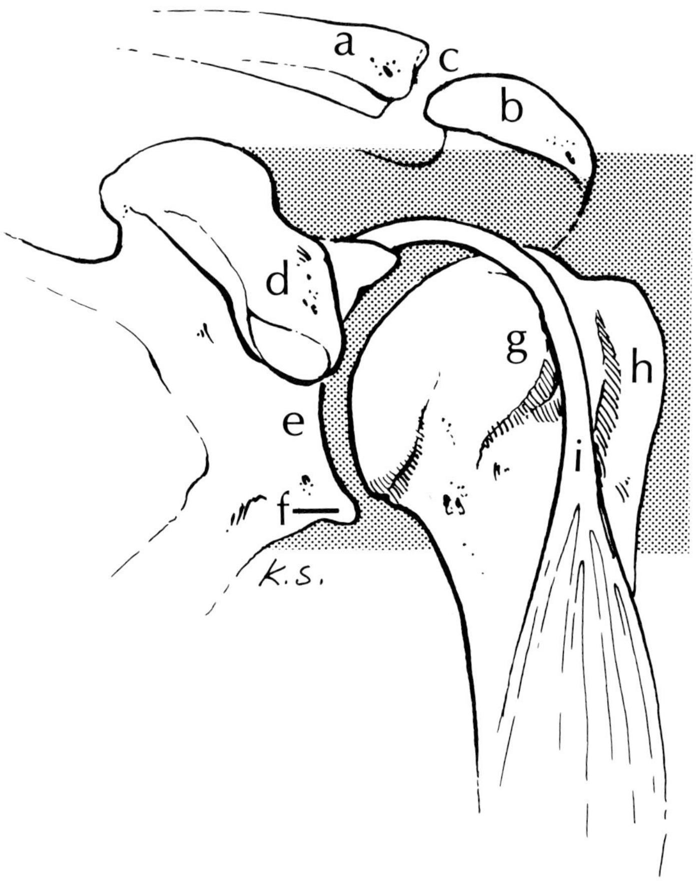

a-clavicle
b- acromion
c-acromioclavicular joint
d-coracoid
e-glenoid
f-labrum
g-lesser tuberosity of humerus
h-greater tuberosity of humerus
i-biceps tendon (long head)

DEVELOPMENT ABNORMALITIES

Abnormalities of the Humerus

1. Aplasia of the humeral head is usually associated with abnormalities of the glenoid.
2. Congenital retroversion, excessive internal rotation of the humeral head leads to recurrent posterior subluxation.
3. The bicipital groove may be too shallow leading to tendon subluxation or too deep leading to restriction of movement of the tendon.

Abnormalities of the Gleno-Humeral Joint

1. Congenital dislocation due to developmental weakness of the capsule or abnormal developmment of the humeral head.

FUNCTIONAL ANATOMY

The shoulder mechanism includes the shoulder girdle (chapter 6) and the glenohumeral joint. These are functionally interdependent, allowing the arms and hands to be positioned through an extensive overlapping area. This mobility is achieved at the expense of stability and recurrent dislocations of the shoulder can occur.

The Joint

Diagram 29. Shoulder anatomy.

The glenohumeral joint is incongruous with a shallow concave glenoid fossa deepened and enlarged by a fibrocartilagenous ring, the glenoid labrum. The convex humeral head is three times larger than the glenoid. The non-articular part of the proximal humerus has two tuberosities separated by the bicipital groove. The greater tuberosity is lateral and the lesser is anteromedial. The articular surface of the humeral head is covered superiorly by the acromion and the coraco-acromial arch but the tuberosities are not covered, they project anterolaterally.

Ligaments

The capsule attaches around the perimeter of the glenoid labrum and the anatomical neck of the humerus. It is loose, allowing an extensive range of motion.

The glenohumeral ligament reinforces the anterior capsule and joins the lesser tuberosity to the anterior edge of the glenoid. It has three bands in a "Z" shape that restrict external rotation when the arm is hanging. An opening between the superior and middle band is often found when the shoulder dislocates anteriorly.

The coraco-humeral ligament joins the under surface of the coracoid to the greater and lesser tuberosities. This ligament reinforces the superior capsule amd resists downward distraction.

There is a large bursa that separates the superior surface of the humerus from the under surface of the acromion. This subacromial bursa allows the head of the humerus to rotate under the acromion without friction.

Muscles

Diagram 30. Scapulo-humeral muscles.

The pure shoulder muscles (scapulo-humeral) are the deltoid and the rotator cuff. The muscles of the rotator cuff are the supraspinatus, the infraspinatus, the teres minor and the subscapularis. These muscles combine to produce the rolling, sliding movement of the humeral head on the glenoid as the shoulder abducts.

The latissimus dorsi and the pectoralis major (not shown in diagram) are accessory muscles that join the proximal humerus to the trunk. The latissimus dorsi joins the inner lip of the bicipital groove to the lumbar vertebral spines and the iliac crest. It internally rotates the arm, extends the shoulder, and depresses the shoulder girdle. The pectoralis major internally rotates and adducts the arm and protrudes the shoulder girdle. These two large truncal muscles have their nerve supply from cervical segments even though their origins have migrated caudally.

The biceps and the long head of the triceps join the scapula to the forearm, crossing both the elbow and the shoulder. These muscles exert their main action on the elbow.

30—Scapulohumeral Muscles—Posterior Aspect

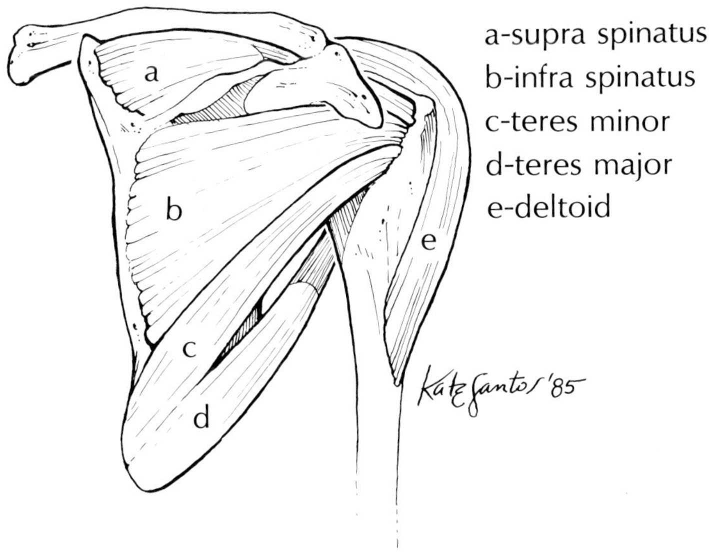

30—Scapulohumeral Muscles—Anterior Aspect

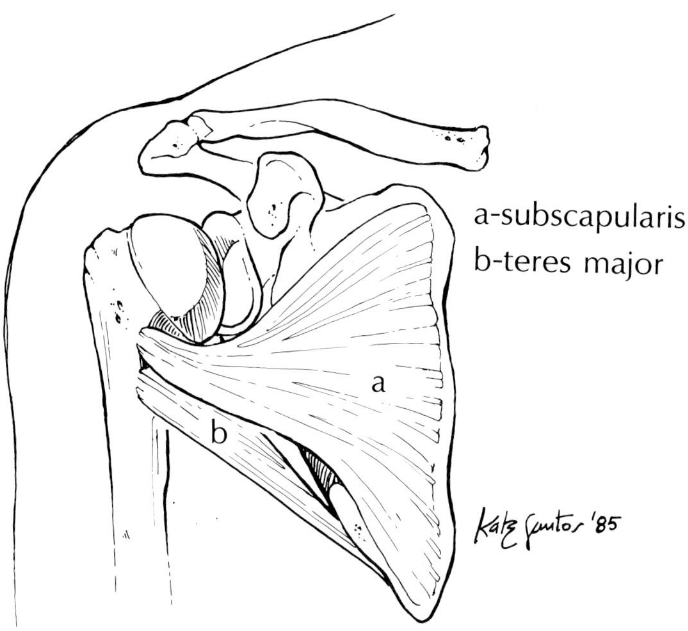

MOVEMENT

Glenohumeral movement requires the complex coordination of the rotator cuff muscles and the deltoid. Abduction of the arm begins with the upward pull of the deltoid and a simultaneous rotation and fixation of the humeral head due to the action of the rotator cuff muscles. The downward pull of the caudal rotator cuff muscles prevents impingement of the greater tuberosity and the coracoacromial arch.

Thus, elevation of the arm from the dependent position to the vertical position requires elevation of the acromion and distal clavicle (upper trapezius), forward rotation of the scapula (serratus anterior) and abduction of the humerus (deltoid and rotator cuff).

At the glenohumeral joint, 120 degrees of abduction occurs and scapular motion contributes the balance (60 degrees).

Internal and external rotation of the glenohumeral joint increases if the arm is abducted to 90 degrees. This relaxes the coraco-humeral ligaments and moves the lesser tuberosity away from the glenoid labrum.

Unlike the hip, which gains stability from the deep acetabulum, the shoulder depends on the ligaments and muscles to support the shallow glenoid.

PHYSICAL EXAMINATION

Examination at Rest

In the relaxed erect position, the arm should hang vertically, resting against the side of the chest. The deltoid muscle creates the rounded contour of the shoulder as it passes over the greater tuberosity laterally and the lesser tuberosity anteriorly. This rounded contour is lost (square shoulder) with an anteromedial dislocation. In this condition, the humeral head can be seen as a prominence below the coracoid and the arm is held in abduction and internal rotation.

31—Shoulder Deformities

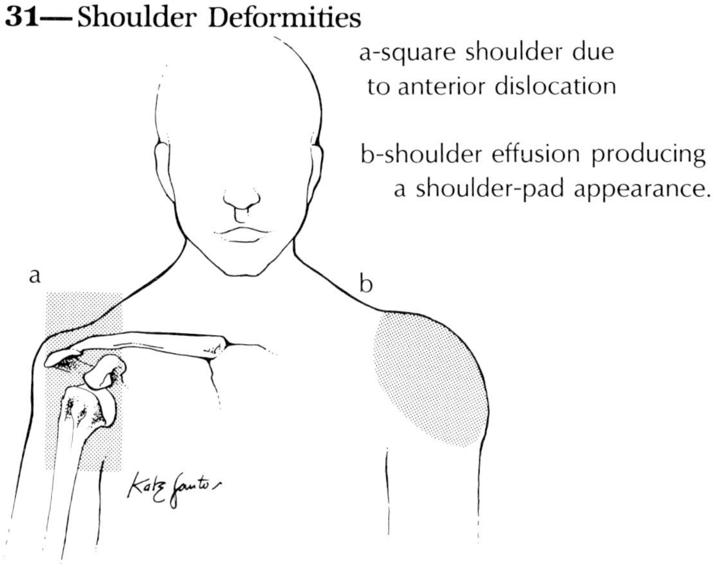

Diagram 31. Shoulder deformities.

Swelling of the scapulo-humeral joint forms a prominence anteriorly, below the coraco-acromial arch and lateral to the coracoid. Atrophy of the deltoid muscle creates a "square shoulder". This differs from a dislocation in that the tuberosities are still visible anterolaterally and the squaring is most marked posteriorly. The supraspinatus muscle should always be examined for atrophy.

Examination with Movement

Figure 6. Total shoulder elevation.
Figure 7. External rotation.
Figure 8. Internal rotation.

Shoulder movement should be examined from the front or the back and both shoulders should be moved simultaneously. A loss of range is usually evident in the movement of total shoulder elevation. Rotation (hands behind head or back) and horizontal flexion (hand on opposite shoulder) will demonstrate whether the restriction is universal or selective.

The kinetics of shoulder movement are of particular diagnostic importance. The rotator cuff is compressed against the under surface of the acromion during the mid arc of abduction (60-120 degrees). The acromioclavicular joint is stressed in the superior arc (120-180 degrees).

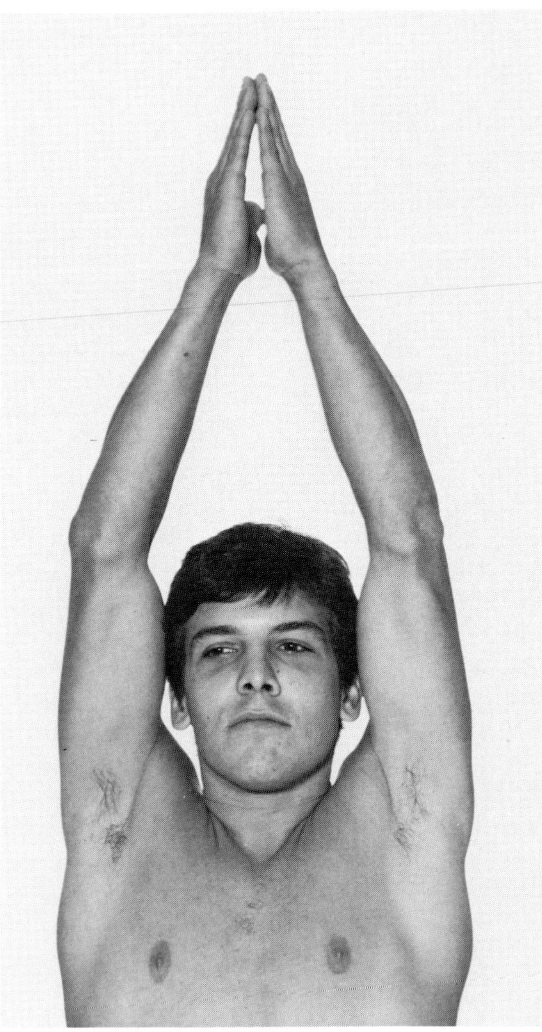

Figure 6

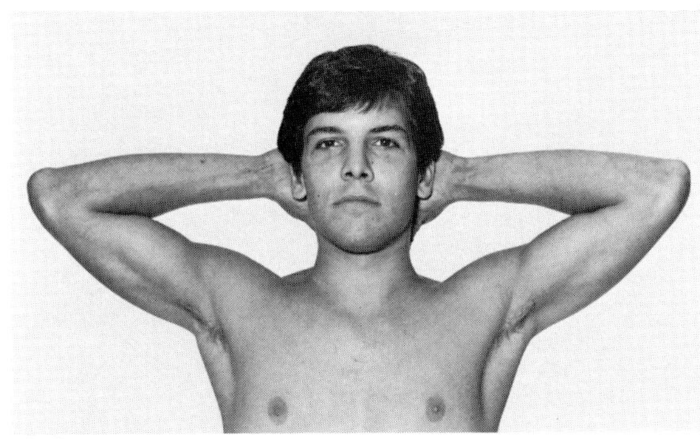

Figure 7

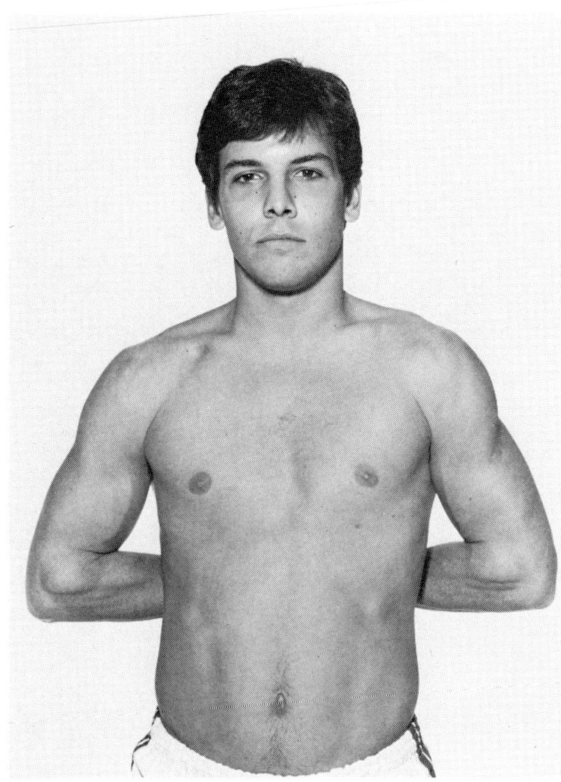

Figure 8

32— Shoulder Examination Position

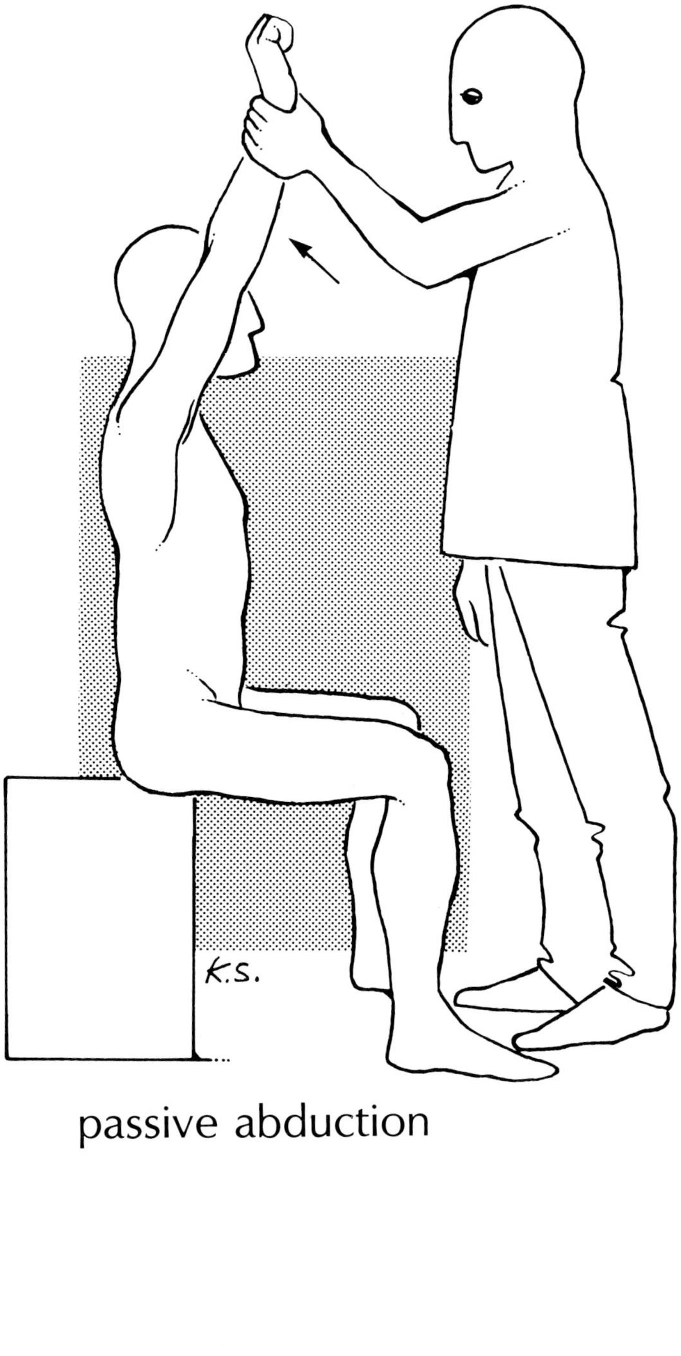

passive abduction

Guarded or interrupted movement in the superior arc suggests acromioclavicular joint disease and guarded or interrupted movement in the mid arc suggests rotator cuff disease.

Mid arc pain may be decreased by abducting with the arm in the externally rotated, or the 'palm up' position or by elevating the arm anteriorly (sagittal flexion). Both of these techniques lessen the impingement of the greater tuberosity against the acromion.

A common trick movement to lessen mid arc pain is to swing the arm up to 80 degrees and then bend the trunk quickly toward the abducting arm. This flexes the glenoid on the humerus without the use of the shoulder muscles. The arm is then stabilized and the trunk straightened.

Palpation

Active Assisted and Passive Movement

Diagram 32. The position for examining the shoulder.

If active movements are restricted or painful, active assisted and passive movements should be tested. This is best done with the patient seated and the examiner standing along side. Palpation of the scapula during passive movement will allow one to judge whether restriction is occurring in the shoulder or the shoulder girdle.

The arm should be abducted in both the coronal and sagittal planes to determine if there is selective stress pain. With the shoulder abducted to 90 degrees and the elbow bent to 90 degrees, the arm is rotated externally (up) and internally (down). The arm is then flexed horizontally across the anterior chest so that the patient's hand rests on the opposite shoulder and finally it is taken down and backward until vertical extension is complete (the racing dive position).

Power failure (restricted active/normal passive range), stress pain and the nature of the end point of restricted range should be noted.

Diagnostic Palpation

The shoulder should be palpated from the front. First, the coracoid is located below the lateral clavicle. Palpating laterally, one can identify the lesser tuberosity, the bicipital groove, the greater tuberosity, and the tip of the acromion. Just lateral to the acromion, one can feel the upper surface of the greater tuberosity where the rotator cuff inserts. The axilla should be palpated for soft tissue masses and tenderness.

Palpation should establish that the humeral head is correctly located lateral to the coracoid. Capsular swelling can be defined anteriorly over the humeral head. Effusions may be moved back and forth under the acromion by gentle anterior and posterior syessure.

The bicipital groove should be palpated for tenderness. Rotation of the arm in the hanging position may cause an unstable bicipital tendon to slip in and out of the groove.

One can accentuate pain arising from the rotator cuff or the subacromial bursa by gently compressing the shoulder during passive abduction. The examiner places one hand on the acromion and the other under the flexed elbow and then gently compresses while passively abducting. If the pain occurs only in a limited position, it suggests that the site of origin is a localized lesion of the rotator cuff.

Cartilagenous or bony crepitus may be palpable over the clavicle if the acromioclavicular joint is damaged. Crepitus will be palpable in the humerus if the glenohumeral joint is damaged. Crepitus will be palpable over the scapula in both conditions.

32— (continued)

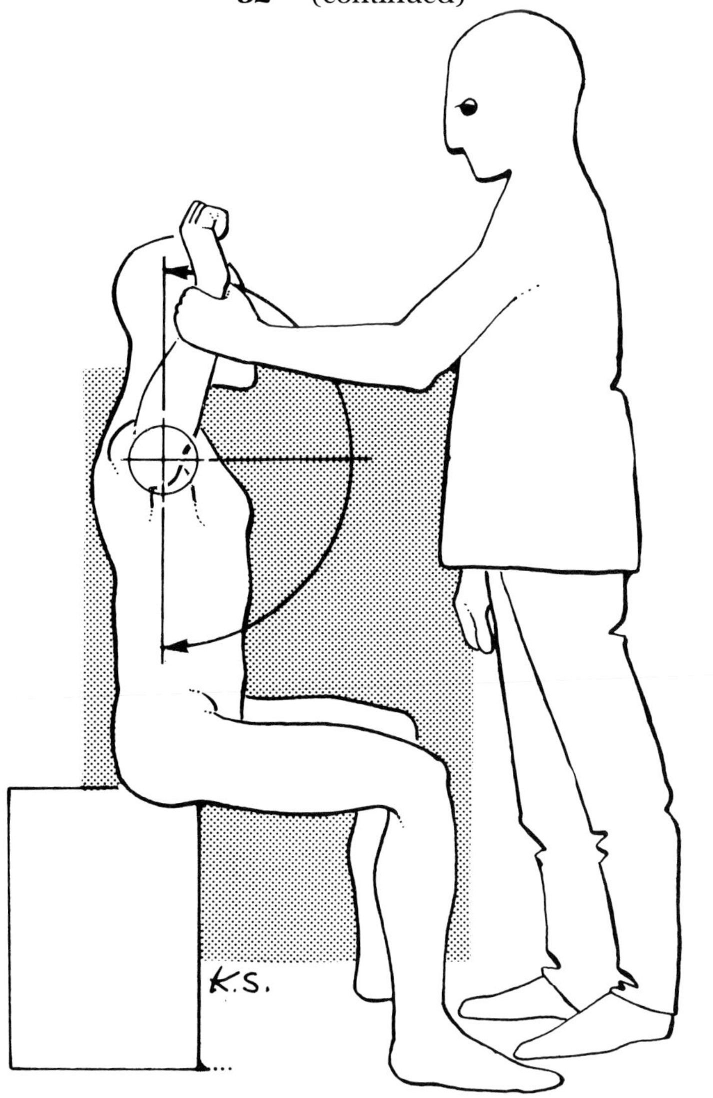

passive rotation,with the elbow flexed to 90°.The examiner may need to support the patient's elbow as well.

8

The Elbow

Abraham Chaiton

DEVELOPMENT

The upper limb bud bends forward to form the elbow during the 5th–6th week. Growth continues at the distal humeral epiphysis until the 17th year and the growth plates of the radial head and olecranon close 12–24 months later.

DEVELOPMENTAL ABNORMALITIES

1. Cubitus varus—Inward deviation of the forearm.
2. Cubitus valgus—Outward deviation of the forearm (Turner's Syndrome).

THE RHEUMATOLOGICAL PHYSICAL EXAMINATION
ISBN 0-8089-1824-9

FUNCTIONAL ANATOMY

The elbow has two joints in a single capsule. The humero-ulnar joint is a modified hinge that allows flexion and extension. The proximal radio-ulnar joint is a pivot joint that participates in pronation and supination of the forearm.

Diagram 33. Anatomy of the elbow.

Bones and Joints

Both the humeral and the ulnar articulations are angled forward 45 degrees, which allows the hinge to close completely and to open to 180 degrees. The humeral trochlea has a groove that accomodates a ridge on the ulnar trochlear notch. This ridge/groove is spiralled so that the elbow angles laterally a few degrees with extension and becomes parallel to the humerus with flexion. The capitulum is spheroid. The anterior and distal surfaces are covered with cartilage.

The proximal ulna has the coronoid process anterior and the olecranon posterior to the trochlear notch. On the infero-lateral lip of the notch is a small concave depression that articulates with the radial head.

The proximal radius has a button shaped head. The proximal surface is concave to articulate with the capitulum and the circumference of this button is flattened to spin on the radial notch of the ulna.

Ligaments

The annular ligament surrounds the radial head, holding it against the radial notch of the ulna, allowing free rotation. The inner surface of the annular ligament is lined by articular cartilage.

The elbow has strong collateral ligaments. The lateral (radial) collateral ligament attaches the annular ligament to the humeral epicondyle and to the ulna. The combined support of the collateral and the annular ligament resists trac-

33—The Elbow

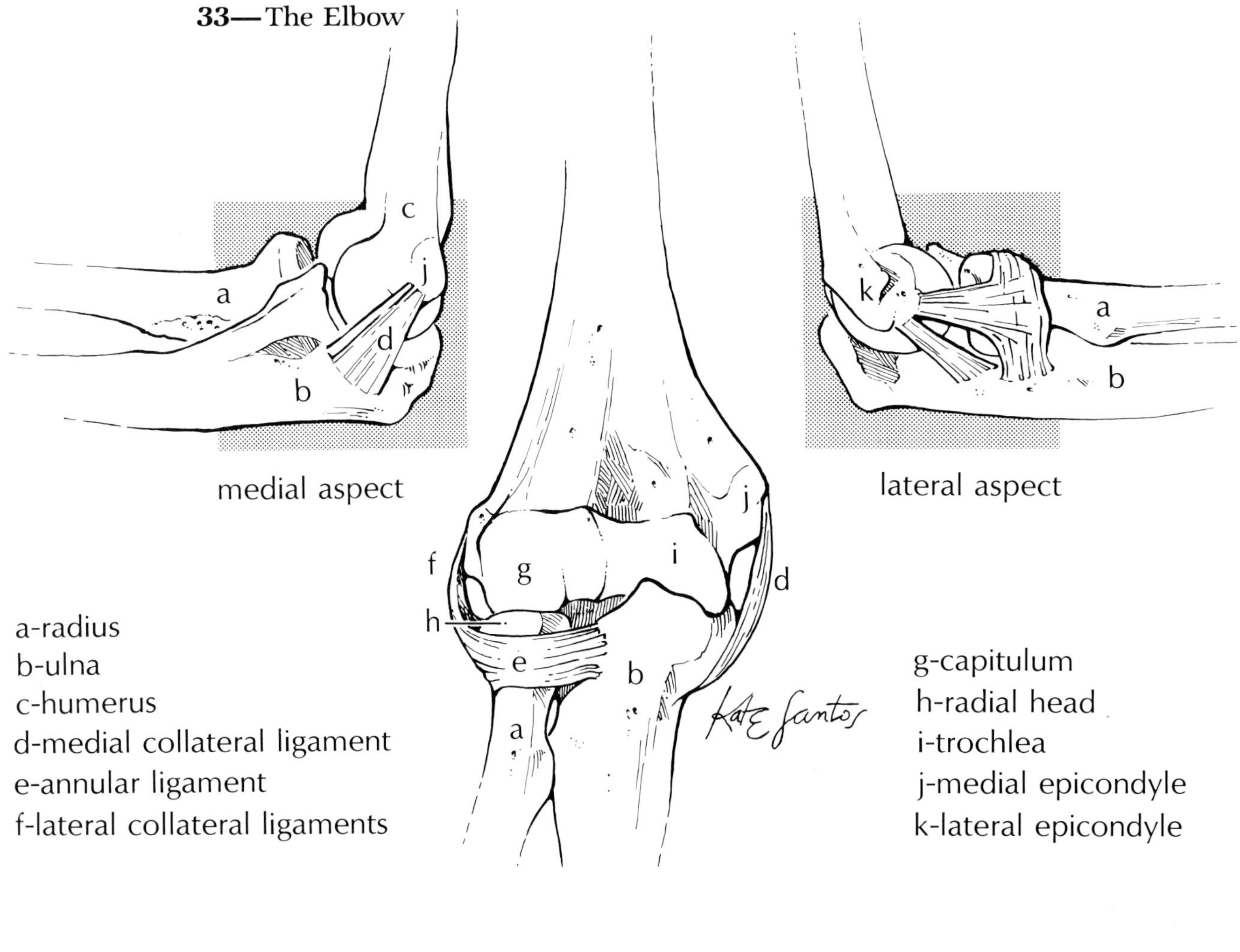

medial aspect

lateral aspect

a-radius
b-ulna
c-humerus
d-medial collateral ligament
e-annular ligament
f-lateral collateral ligaments

g-capitulum
h-radial head
i-trochlea
j-medial epicondyle
k-lateral epicondyle

tion on the radius. The medial (ulnar) collateral ligament is fan shaped, attaching the medial epicondyle to the medial edge of the trochlear notch.

Muscles

There are three flexor muscles at the elbow. The biceps and the brachioradialis are long and the brachialis is short. The biceps joins the scapula to the bicipital tuberosity of the radius. This tuberosity projects medially from the proximal neck of the radius so that the biceps acts as a powerful supinator of the forearm as well as a flexor of the elbow. The brachioradialis joins the lateral supra-condylar ridge of the humerus to the radial styloid. The brachialis joins the anterior surface of the lower humerus to the coronoid process of the ulna.

The triceps is an extensor muscle with three heads. The long head originates at the infra glenoid tubercle of the scapula, the two short heads originate from the back of the humerus above and below the spiral groove. They combine to insert into the posterior surface of the olecranon.

MOVEMENTS

The hinging movement of the elbow allows 145 degrees of active flexion from the fully extended position. Passive flexion can usually achieve another 10–15 degrees when the muscles are relaxed. The elbow hyperextends 10 degrees in many normal women. Heavily muscled individuals may lack 10 degrees at both ends of range.

The limit to flexion is impingement of the soft tissues of the arm and forearm. Extension is limited by the anterior capsule and by impingement of the olecranon against the humerus.

PHYSICAL EXAMINATION

The proximal and distal radio-ulnar joints will be considered in the next chapter.

Inspection at Rest

Shape

In the extended supinated position the elbow angles laterally, 5–10 degrees in the male and up to 20 degrees in the female.

Size

Diagram 34. Swellings at the elbow.

Swelling in the joint capsule causes a prominence around the radial head. This is the most superficial part of the joint. Localized swelling in the olecranon bursa is noted under and slightly behind the olecranon. Subcutaneous rheumatoid nodules on the posterior surface of the proximal ulna may coexist with an olecranon bursitis or may resemble one.

34—Swellings at the Elbow

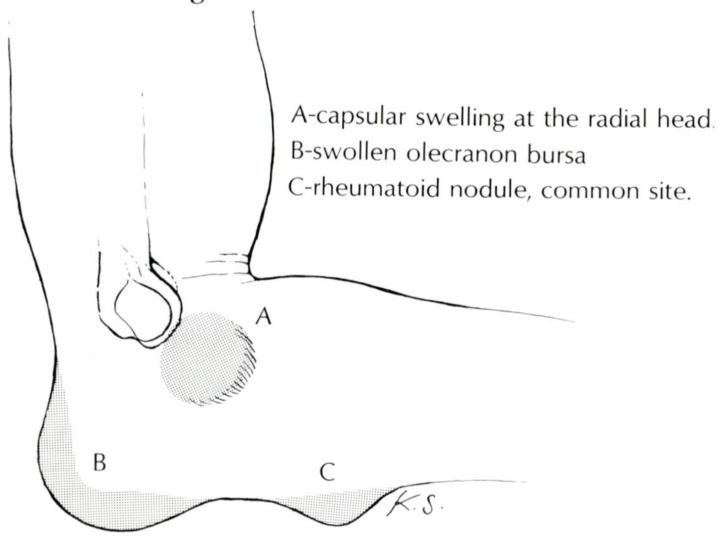

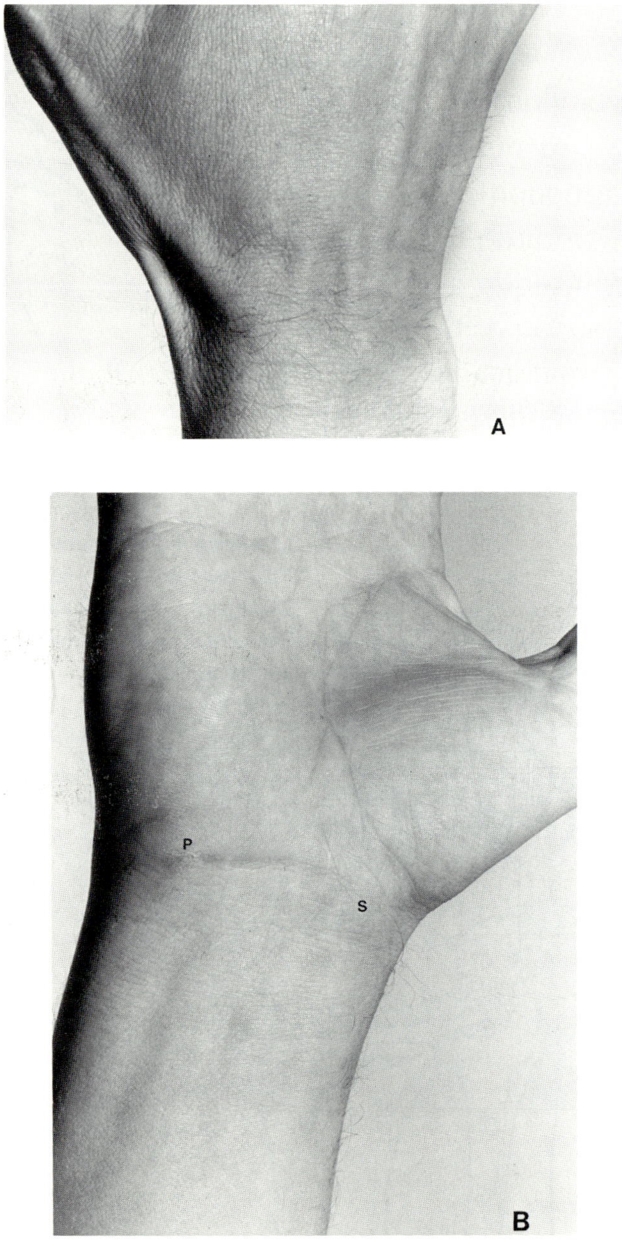

Figure 36

PHYSICAL EXAMINATION

Inspection at Rest

With the hand in the prone resting position the dorsal prominence of the ulnar head can be seen. Distal to the ulnar head is a steep slope. Radially, Lister's tubercle forms a prominence at the mid point of the distal radius. Distal to this prominence is a hollow bounded by the extensor indicis on the ulnar side and the extensor carpi radialis brevis on the radial side. On the radial side of the wrist is another hollow, the "anatomical snuff box". This is a depression between the tendon of extensor pollicis longus and the more radial extensor pollicis brevis and abductor pollicis longus.

Figure 36. (A & B) To show surface anatomy of the wrist.

On the flexor side of the wrist two prominences can be seen at the proximal palmar crease. On the radial side is the tubercle of the scaphoid (s) and on the ulnar side is the pisiform bone (p). When the wrist is flexed, a particularly deep horizontal crease develops about 1 cm. proximal to the palm. This is the level of the volar margin of the radio carpal joint.

Diagram 41. Axis of wrist and hand.

With the hand and arm at rest, the longitudinal axis of the radius and the 2nd metacarpal are in line. Habitual deviations from this line should be described as radial or ulnar posturing. The dorsal surface of the 3rd metacarpal should be in approximately the same plane as the dorsal surface of the distal radius with the wrist in the neutral position. A common deformity in rheumatoid disease is volar subluxation and shortening at the carpus. If marked, a visible step can be seen at the radio carpal joint. (See Figure 31.)

Diagram 42. Deformities at the wrist.

Swelling of the wrist is visible on the dorsum. If confined to the wrist joint, the swelling fills the hollows distal to the radius and ulna, and may distend them. Swelling of the extensor tendon sheaths extends proximal to the joint line and shows longitudinal grooves that correspond to the attachments of the extensor retinaculum to the underlying bone.

Healed fractures of the distal radius change the orientation of the wrist and may simulate swelling. This is particularly true if the distal fragment heals with dorsal angulation, the so-called "dinner fork" deformity of a Colles fracture.

Much information can gleaned from a few simple observations. The bulk of the forearm musculature indicates strength or its absence while the thickness of the keratin layer of the palm speaks clearly of the amount of loading the palm is subject to.

41—Axis of the Wrist and Hand

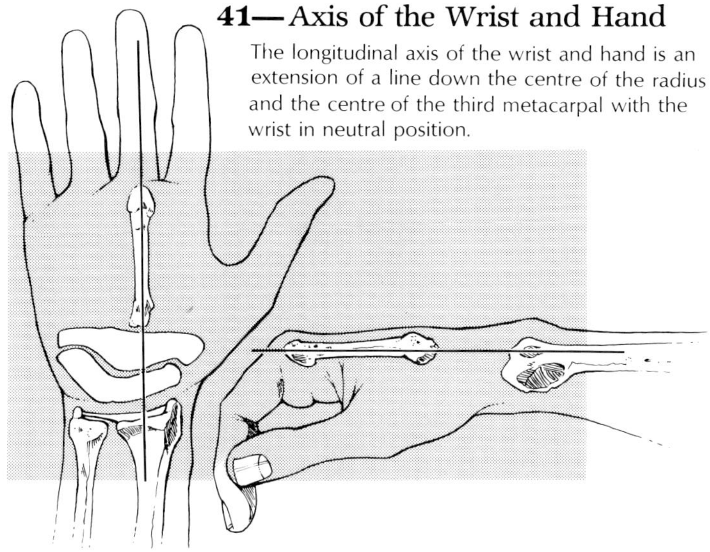

The longitudinal axis of the wrist and hand is an extension of a line down the centre of the radius and the centre of the third metacarpal with the wrist in neutral position.

42—Deformities at the Wrist

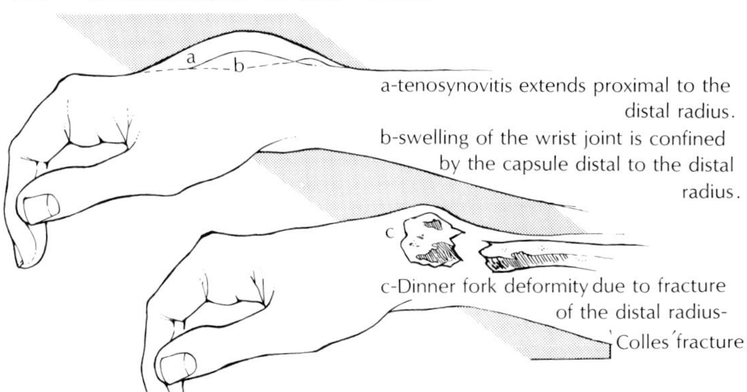

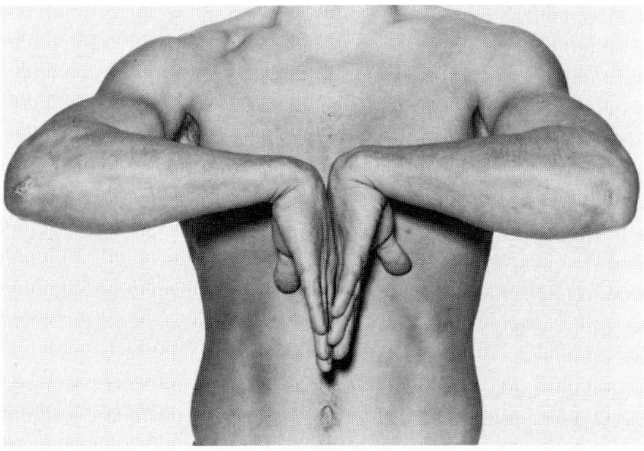

Figure 13

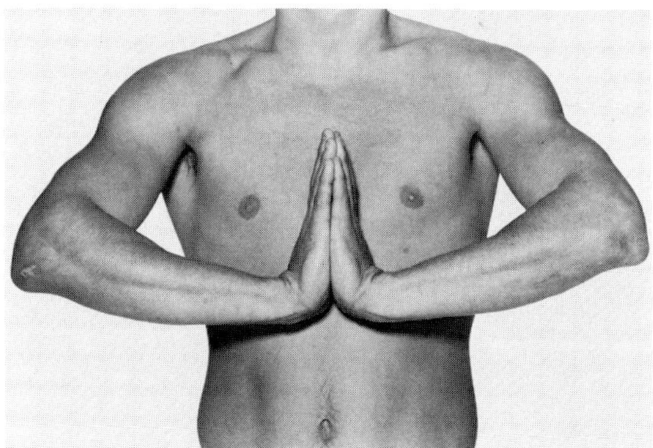

Figure 14

Inspection with Movement

Figure 13. Wrist flexion
Figure 14. Wrist extension

The range of movement in all planes should be inspected for restriction. Using the combined active and passive technique illustrated in the photographs, most adults will flex and extend to 90 degrees or slightly greater. Those individuals who do heavy manual work and have a thick boned physique may lack 10–15 degrees and still be normal.

Normally, wrist extension is not limited by the long flexor tendons. However, a flexor tenosynovitis may limit wrist extension unless the fingers are allowed to flex. This can be achieved by allowing the fingers to interlace when the wrist is pushed into extension.

Guarding can be recognized by noting the reluctance of the patient to push the hands together firmly.

Palpation

Active Assisted and Passive Movements

As with other joints, the wrist should be tested for power failure (restricted active/normal passive range). Tethering or blocking is inferred from the nature of the end point of restricted passive range. Stress pain is noted.

Diagnostic Palpation

Structural Identification

Each carpal bone is identifiable by palpation. The thumb, ring and little metacarpals move at the carpo-metacarpal joints. This movement allows one to identify the trapezium proximal to the thumb and the hamate proximal to the little and ring. The bases of the index and middle metacarpals can be identified by the prominent exostoses associated with the insertions of the extensor carpi radialis tendons. Just proximal to these prominences are the subadjacent trapezoid and capitate.

The triquetrum is readily identified by feeling just distal to the prominence of the ulnar head. The lunate is elusive. Fortunately, the long axis of the third metacarpal, projected proximally, passes very close to the scapho-lunate junction with the wrist in neutral. Thus, the lunate can be felt just distal to the radial rim at the ulnar side of this axis and made more prominent by 10-15 degrees of wrist flexion. The scaphoid can be felt on the radial side of this same axis.

As each bone is identified, they should be grasped individually between finger and thumb and differential motion attempted. Significant instability is abnormal.

Angulation and translocation are determined by defining the dorsal surface of the 3rd metacarpal. It should be on the same plane as the dorsal surface of the radius. One can passively angle the 3rd metacarpal 15 degrees radially and 35 degrees ulnarly from the long axis of the radius. Both the resting position and the range of deviation from that position should be measured to describe angulation accurately.

Diagram 43. Carpal collapse.

Loss of carpal height can be estimated by comparing the distance from the base of the 3rd metacarpal to the distal radius in the neutral position to the length of the 3rd metacarpal. The ratio of carpal height/metacarpal length should be about 1/2. Generally, the carpal height in the neutral position will admit the tips of the patient's index and middle fingers

Diagram 44. Tuck sign.

Swelling of the extensor tendon sheaths moves with the tendons. Thus, when the fingers are actively extended the distal margin of the swelling moves proximally and folds in, like a sheet being tucked under the mattress (the tuck sign). Extensor tendons are normally definable over the wrist, tenosynovitis obscures that definition. Pain on resisted finger extension indicates tenosynovitis.

Swelling of the wrist joint will lift the tendons and fill in the normal hollows. When there is a tenosynovitis as well, wrist swelling is difficult to establish. The wrist joint cannot be palpated from the flexor side due to the overlying tendons. Flexor tenosynovitis can be noted as swelling proximal to the carpal tunnel (i.e. proximal to the palm).

Tenderness should be localized. Particular attention should be paid to the retinacular tunnel of the extensor pollicis brevis and abductor pollicis longus on the lateral side of the distal radius just proximal to the "anatomical snuff box". This area is tender in stenosing tenosynovitis of De Quervain. Tendinous stress pain can be elicited in the same area in this condition by having the patient grasp the thumb and ulnarly deviate the wrist (Finkelstein's sign).

Percussion tenderness of the flexor retinaculum associated with paraesthesias in the median nerve distribution is a sign of carpal tunnel syndrome (Tinel's sign). Phalen's test (sustained acute flexion of the wrist) usually brings on incipient carpal tunnel symptoms within 30 seconds. If the wrist cannot be flexed, an alternative method is to apply direct pressure over the median nerve (just radial to the palmaris longus tendon at the wrist) and sustain the pressure for 30 seconds.

43—Carpal Collapse

The height of the carpus a-should be equal to half the length of the third metacarpal b. Less than half indicates carpal collapse.

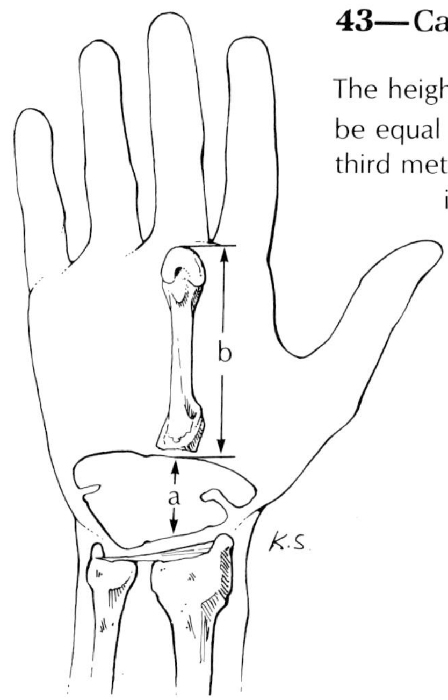

44—The Tuck Sign— Extensor Tenosynovitis at the Wrist

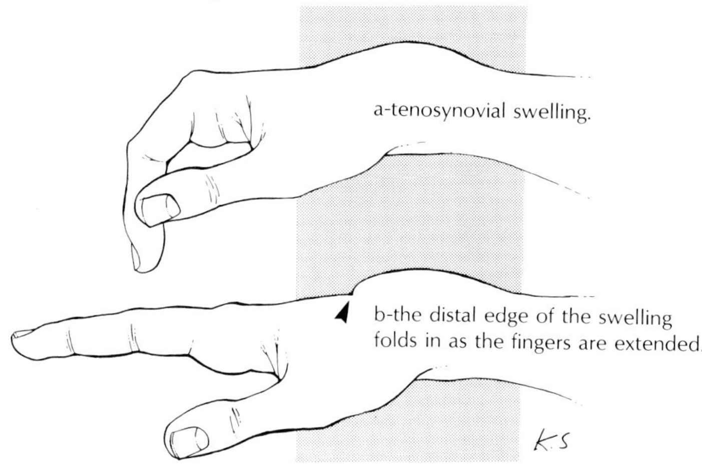

11
The Hand

Robert Y. McMurtry

The hand has two primary functions. It is the principal sensory organ of touch and it is uniquely specialized for grasping. The radial side of the hand performs pinch-grip between fingers and thumb. The ulnar side of the hand performs power-grip between fingers and palm. It is this remarkably adaptable structure that has enabled man to manipulate the environment.

DEVELOPMENT

The discoid distal limb bud develops five cartilagenous rays in the early embryonic period. These rays separate into fingers and segment into metacarpals and phalanges during the late embryonic period (6th–8th week). At birth the hand is short and broad. The length of the fingers, relative to the metacarpals increases to maturity.

THE RHEUMATOLOGICAL PHYSICAL EXAMINATION
ISBN 0-8089-1824-9

45—Bones of the Hand

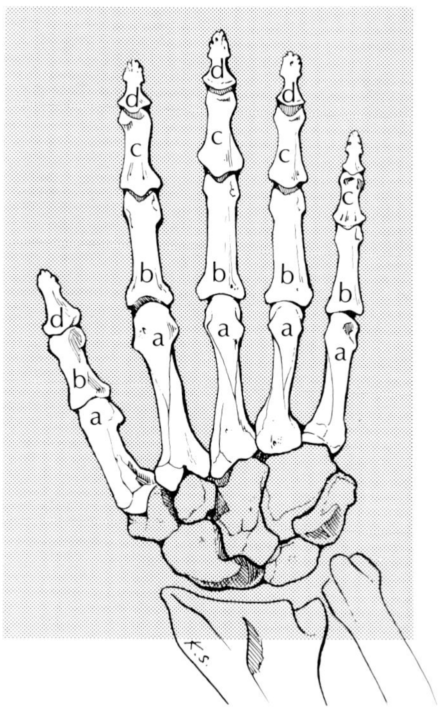

a-metacarpals
b-proximal phalanges
c-middle phalanges
d-distal phalanges

DEVELOPMENTAL ABNORMALITIES OF THE HANDS

These are common and may occur as an isolated defect or as part of an extensive developmental abnormality.

1. Absence of the whole hand
2. Absence of the central rays—Lobster claw, mirror hands
3. Supernumerary Rays—polydactyly, polyphalangy
4. Failure of separation—syndactyly
5. Arrested development—brachydactyly
6. Excessive growth—megalodactyly

FUNCTIONAL ANATOMY

Diagram 45. Bones of the hand.

The bony structure of the hand is relatively simple. Five rays, composed of a series of small bones, extend out from the carpus. The first ray (thumb) has three bones. The rest have four. The bones get smaller distally.

The carpo-metacarpal (CMC) joint of the thumb is very mobile. The distal surface of the trapezium is shaped like a saddle. The metacarpal of the thumb, like a horseman, sits on the saddle facing the little finger. The CMC joint allows the thumb to rock forward and back in the saddle, to sway from side to side and to twist axially during opposition.

The 2nd and 3rd CMC joints are rigid. The 4th and 5th are mobile but less so than the thumb. The distal surface of the hamate has two articular concavities to accommodate the bases of the 4th and 5th metacarpals, allowing them to flex forward toward the thumb thus creating the hollow of the palm.

The metacarpo-phalangeal (MCP) joints are modified hinges. The metacarpals have rounded ends. The base of the proximal phalanges are concave and small but each has a cartilagenous extension on the volar side called the palmar plate.

The interphalangeal (IP) joints are true hinges. The proximal surface of the IP joint has two slightly elevated condyles separated by a groove. The distal surface of the IP joint has a central ridge separating two hollows. The IP joints have a palmar plate similar to the MCP joints. The bicondylar structure plus snug collateral ligaments prevent significant rotation or lateral flexion at the IP joint.

Ligaments

The CMC joints are supported by simple capsular ligaments. The MCP joints have eccentric collateral ligaments that tighten only in full flexion. In the extended position the collateral ligaments are loose, allowing abduction, adduction, and rotation, similar to a ball and socket joint. In the flexed position the collateral ligaments become tight, preventing angulation or rotation.

Diagram 46. Collateral ligaments of MCP and IP joints.

The collateral ligaments of the IP joints are centrally placed and remain taut in all positions. Volar extensions of the collateral ligaments support the volar plate and keep it in contact with the rounded proximal bony surface.

The deep transverse metacarpal ligament joins the volar plates of the MCP joints 2–5. Fibrous tunnels are present on the volar aspect of the proximal and middle phalanges of all the fingers and on the metacarpal and proximal phalanx of the thumb. These tunnels hold the flexor tendons and their synovial sheaths.

46—Collateral Ligaments of the MCP and IP Joints

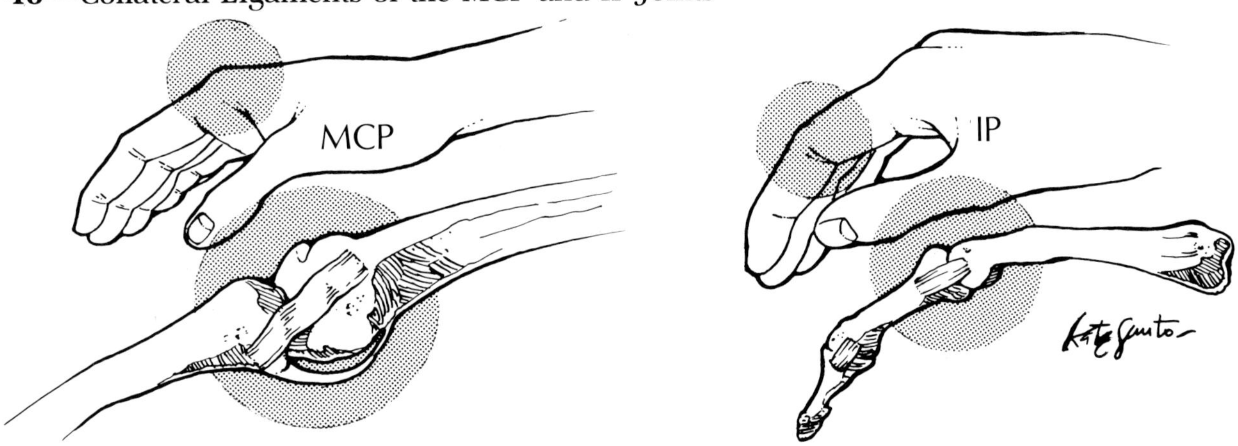

The collateral ligaments tighten in flexion and loosen in extension.

The collateral ligaments remain tight in Both flexion and extension.

47— Palmar Flexor Retinaculum

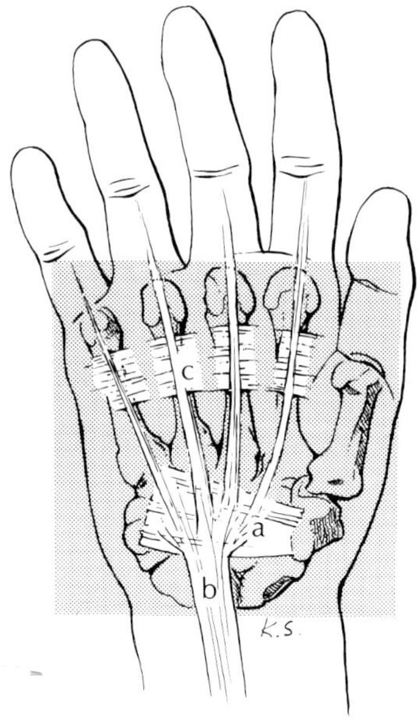

a- flexor retinaculum

b-palmaris longus

c-palmar fascial strands extend to digits with attachments to skin and transverse metacarpal ligament.

48— Flexor Tendon Sheaths of the Hand

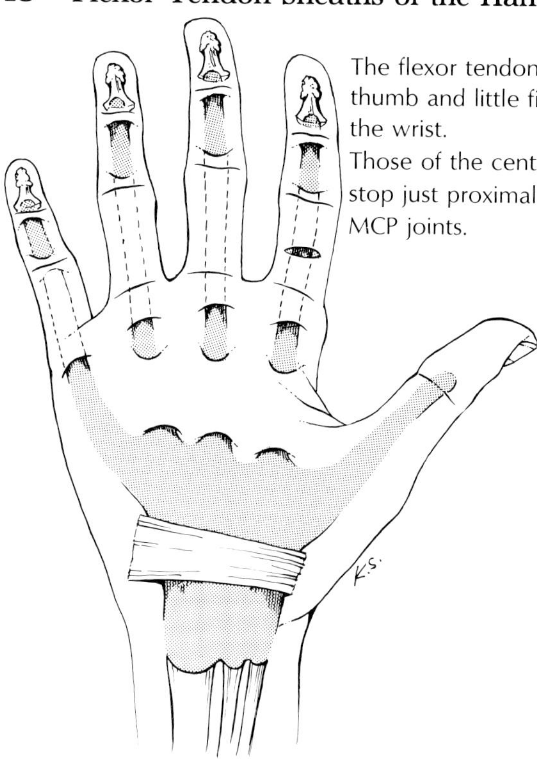

The flexor tendon sheath of the thumb and little finger extend to the wrist.
Those of the central three rays stop just proximal to the MCP joints.

Diagram 47. Palmar fascia and flexor retinaculum.

The palmar fascia is not a ligament. It is an extension of the palmaris longus tendon that partly inserts into the flexor retinaculum and partly divides into four longitudinal bundles that run through the subcutaneous tisssue superficial to the flexor tendons. In the distal part of the palm the bands divide into a deep portion that attaches to the sides of the volar plate and a superficial portion that extends distally to insert into the proximal and distal phalanx. The skin of the palm is firmly attached to the palmar fascia by many short bands.

Muscles and Tendons

There are twenty seven muscles that govern hand movements. Nine of the hand muscles are extrinsic, i.e. their origins and muscle bellies are in the forearm, influencing the hand by long tendons. The 18 intrinsic muscles of the hand are located on the palmar surface and in the interspaces between the metacarpal bones. The interaction of these muscles, which results in the complexity of hand function, is beyond the scope of this text.

The extrinsic muscles flex and extend the fingers and thumb. The intrinsic muscles hollow the palm, adduct and abduct the MCP joints, and assist in flexion of the MCP and extension of the IP joints.

Diagram 48. Flexor tendon sheaths.

Where the flexor tendons pass through fibrous tunnels they are enclosed in synovial sheaths. The synovial sheaths of the 5th finger and the thumb are continuous with the radial and ulnar bursa at the carpal tunnel. The sheaths for the 2nd, 3rd, and 4th rays begin just proximal to the MCP joint and extend distally to the base of the distal phalanx. There are no extensor tendon sheaths distal to the wrist.

Synovial sheaths are found where there are tendon pulleys and their presence, in turn, is determined by the character of motion at the adjacent joint. Thus, at the wrist where both flexion and extension occur, pulleys are essential on the volar and dorsal aspect to prevent bowstringing of the tendons. The hand joints simply flex and extension occurs to neutral only (slightly more at the MCP joints). Accordingly, an elaborate system of pulleys is found on the flexor aspect (with tenosynovium) and neither pulley nor tenosynovium is found on the extensor aspect.

MOVEMENTS

Diagram 49. Postures of the hand.

The thumb CMC joint is tri-axial (moves in three planes). Flexion/extension occurs perpendicular to the nail (40–50 degrees), abduction/adduction parallel to the nail (40 degrees). Rotation occurs during opposition (80 degrees). The MCP joint of the thumb allows 90–100 degrees of flexion/extension and 20 degrees of abduction and 10 degrees of adduction. There is considerable individual variation. The IP joint of the thumb is a hinge but careful observation will reveal 10–15 degrees of pronation (opposition) during flexion.

The index and middle fingers are part of the central fixed unit of the hand together with the distal carpal row. Virtually no motion occurs at the CMC joints. The index MCP joint flexes to 90 degrees and the middle MCP slightly more. They extend just beyond neutral and adduct and abduct in this position.

The ring and little fingers differ from the index and middle in that their CMC joints move. From the neutral position, the ring flexes 15 degrees and the little 30 degrees. This motion is critical for power grip.

All the IP joints of the fingers are similar. The proximal joints flex to 100–110 degrees and the distal joints flex to 85 degrees. Normally they extend only to neutral (180 degrees).

PHYSICAL EXAMINATION OF THE HAND

Inspection at Rest

The dorsum of the hand is covered with thin skin allowing easy identification of the extensor mechanism and the dorsal aspect of the articular structures. The palmar surface is covered by thick skin, subcutaneous tissue, and fascia so that the deeper structures cannot be seen.

49— Postures of the Hand

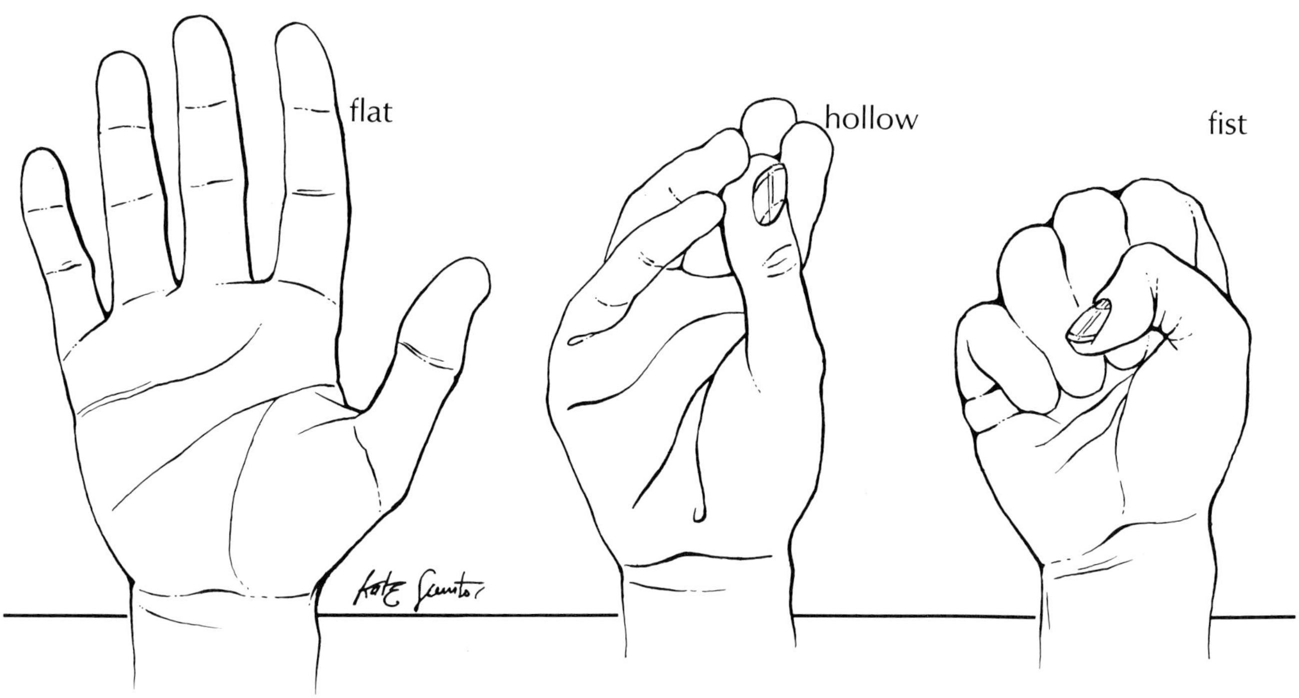

50—Hand Deformities

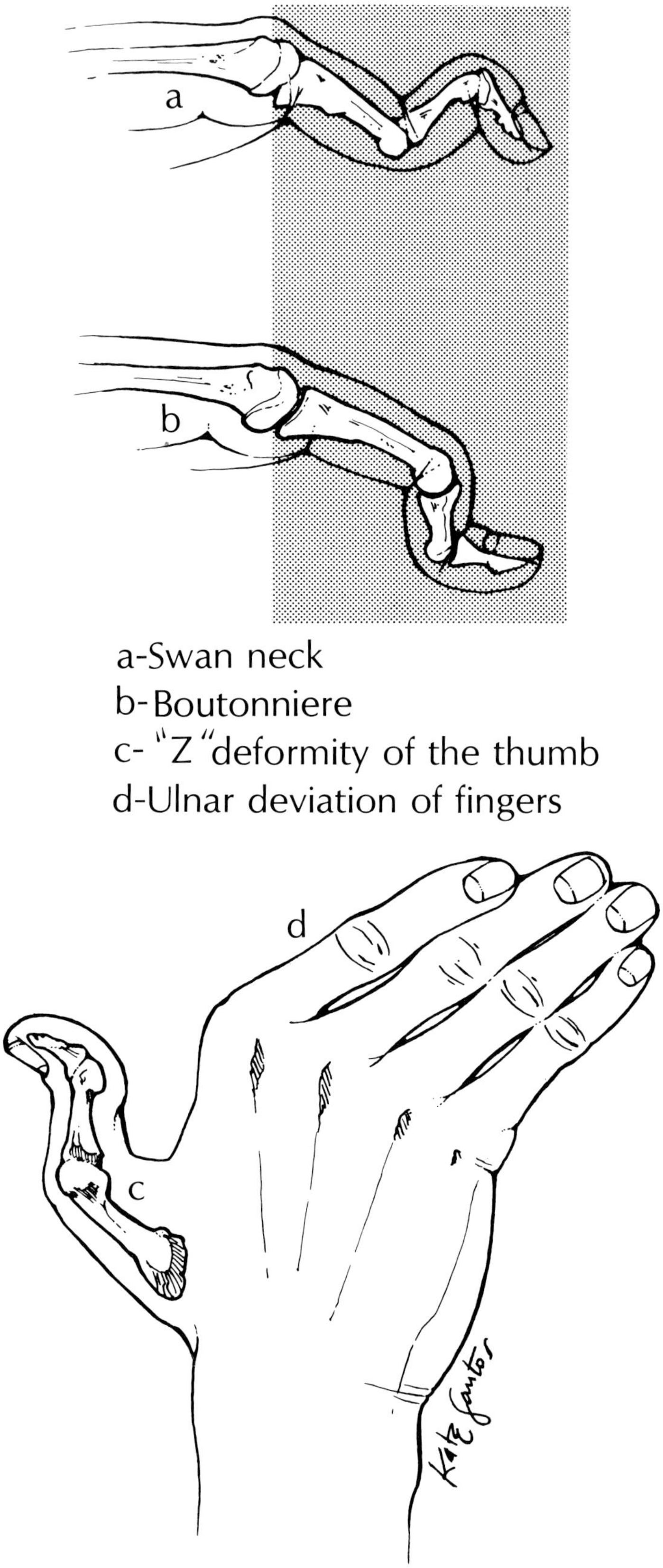

Each digital ray is inspected for deformity. Volar translocation of the finger at the MCP joint must be severe to be visible as a step. Pure rotatory deformities are rare but rotation may be associated with angulation or translocation. Abnormalities of length may be due to prenatal or postnatal developmental deficiencies. Inflammatory conditions like rheumatoid arthritis can lead to marked loss of bone and visible shortening.

Diagram 50. Hand deformities.

The "Boutonniere" deformity is flexion of the proximal IP joint and hyperextension of the distal IP joint of a finger. The "Swan Neck" deformity is hyperextension of the proximal IP joint and flexion of the distal IP joint of the finger. The MCP joints often show an ulnar drift in inflammatory joint disease and the thumb may develop a "Z" deformity with flexion of the MCP joint and hyperextension of the IP joint.

Many deformities can occur. Although the abbreviations, (Z, Boutonniere, Swan Neck) are useful, the beginner would be wise to describe the abnormalities at each joint level.

Each joint is inspected for swelling. Each swelling is inspected to determine if it is confined to the joint capsule or a tendon sheath. If the swellings are multiple the distribution is noted.

The extensor tendons cross the MCP joints at the mid dorsum. If the supporting bands of the extensor expansion are damaged the tendons may slide into the inter-metacarpal valleys where they are clearly visible. This occurs characteristically to the ulnar side.

Muscle groups are inspected for atrophy. The skin of the palm is inspected for thickening of keratin layer, contractures, and scars.

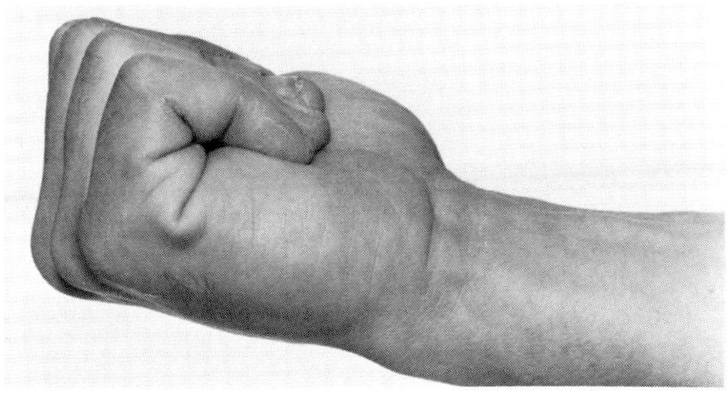
Figure 15

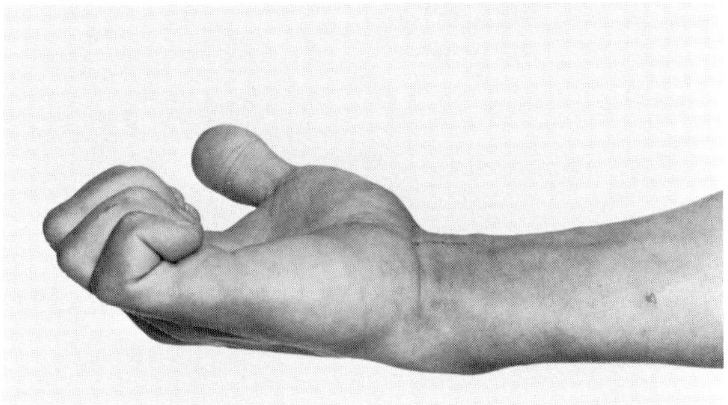
Figure 16

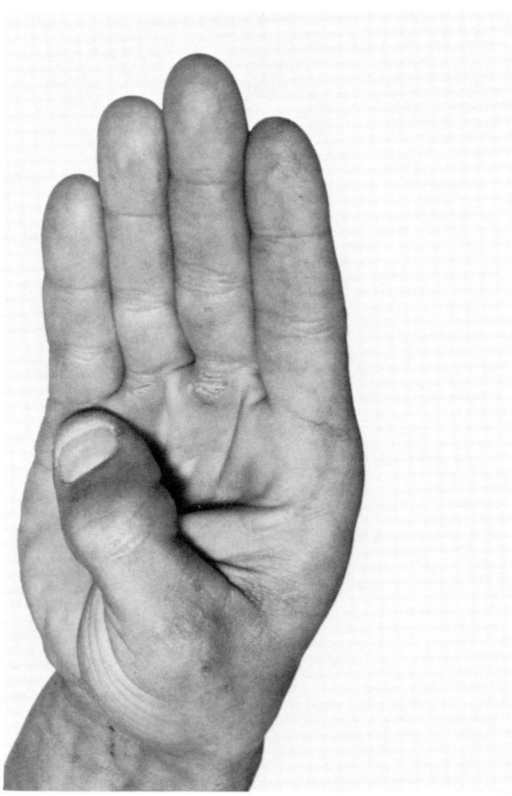

Inspection with Movement

Figure 15. Metacarpophalangeal flexion.
Figure 16. Interphalangeal flexion.
Figure 17. Thumb opposition.

With the hand in the prone position the fingers and thumb are fully extended against gravity. The hand is supinated and the sequence of movements, illustrated above, is performed. This does not test the movement at the 4th and 5th CMC joint but selective loss of these movements is extremely rare.

The range of movement is observed for selective or generalized restriction. The kinetics of movement are observed for guarding, interrupted, or trick movements. A "trigger finger" or thumb is an involuntary hesitation in flexion or extension usually due to the flexor tendon sticking in the tendon sheath. Once the obstruction is past, the movement is free and unrestricted. The "triggering" may be painful.

Palpation

Active Assisted and Passive Movement

As with other joints, the hand should be tested for power failure (restricted active/normal passive range). Tethering or blocking is inferred from the nature of the end point of restricted passive range. Stress pain is noted.

Each finger and each joint is palpated individually. Range of motion and stability is assessed by attempting to produce ulnar deviation, radial deviation, and hyperextension at each IP joint. Instability is present when any of the

51— Bunnell's Test for Intrinsic Tightness

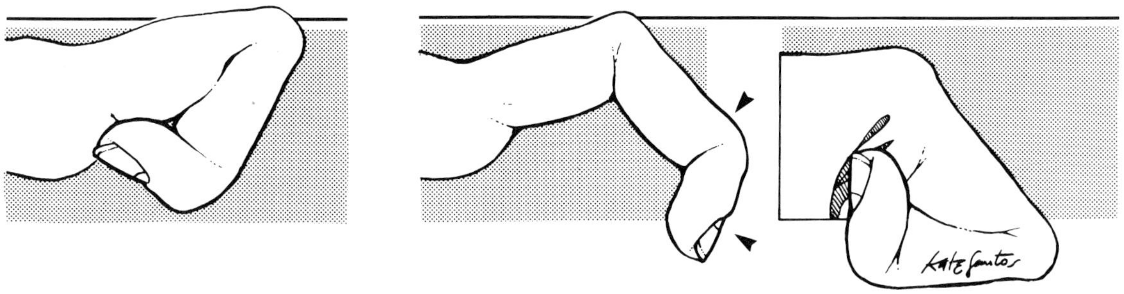

above motions are greater than that of the neighbouring digit or the similar digit of the opposite hand.

Diagram 51. To show Bunnell's test.

Bunnell's Test

The intrinsic muscles may develop contractures inhibiting flexion of the IP joints when the MCP joint is extended.

1. The MCP joint is passively hyperextended and the IP joints are passively flexed. If full flexion is possible the test is negative. If flexion is restricted, the second part of the test is carried out.

2. The MCP joint is passively flexed and the IP joints are passively flexed. If there is a significant increase in IP flexion when the MCP joint is flexed and the intrinsic muscles relaxed, Bunnell's test is positive, indicating an intrinsic contracture.

A refinement of this test is to perform it with the MCP joint in radial or ulnar deviation to selectively stress the opposite intrinsic muscle.

52— Collateral Instability at the MCP Joint

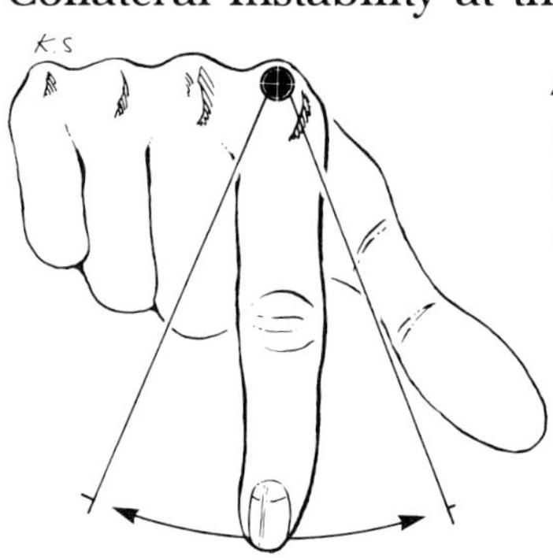

AT 90° flexion the MCP is stable normally.Collateral instability is shown by side to side passive movement in this position.

Diagram 52. MCP collateral stability test.

Test for Collateral Instability of the MCP Joint

The MCP joint is flexed to 90 degrees to tighten the collateral ligaments, then the finger is moved from side to side to test the integrity of the collateral ligaments. If instability is discovered one should note whether it is the radial or the ulnar collateral or both and the extent of the instability should be estimated.

Diagnostic Palpation

Structural Identification

Starting at the distal phalanx of the thumb, the pulp is palpated and then the sides and front and back of the IP joint. Over the proximal phalanx one can feel the long flexor and extensor tendons. The MCP joint of the thumb is large and the two bony sesamoids on the volar surface may be recognizable with the flexor tendon moving between and beneath them.

The dorsum of the first metacarpal is palpable throughout its length and the proximal end is determined by the step down into the "anatomical snuff box". The tendon of the long extensor of the thumb is easily palpable as it angles toward the mid line. The tendon of the short extensor is difficult to separate from the metacarpal. Since the flexor surface of the thumb metacarpal is covered by the muscles of the thenar eminence, the long flexor tendon is difficult to feel proximal to the MCP joint.

The digits are then examined in a manner similar to the thumb. With any of the MCP or IP joints flexed, the convex proximal articular surface should be palpated for erosions, irregularities, or synovial thickening.

Diagram 53. MCP surface anatomy.

Volar subluxation of the proximal phalanx on the metacarpal head can be appreciated if the head remains palpable above the phalanx with the joint in full extension or if it projects beyond the phalanx with the joint in full flexion.

Resisted digital flexion makes the flexor tendons palpable until they enter the carpal tunnel.

Swollen joints are palpated for bony enlargement or capsular distension. If the swelling is soft then 4 fingers are used, 3 to compress the sides and bottom and the 4th to sense the hydraulic lift of the "balloon sign" that signifies an effusion. The swollen joint is palpated in the neutral and flexed position since the intracapsular pressure increases as the joint approaches the limit of range. If the swelling becomes firmer with flexion, it is likely to be intracapsular fluid or synovial hypertrophy.

53—MCP Surface Anatomy

Normal

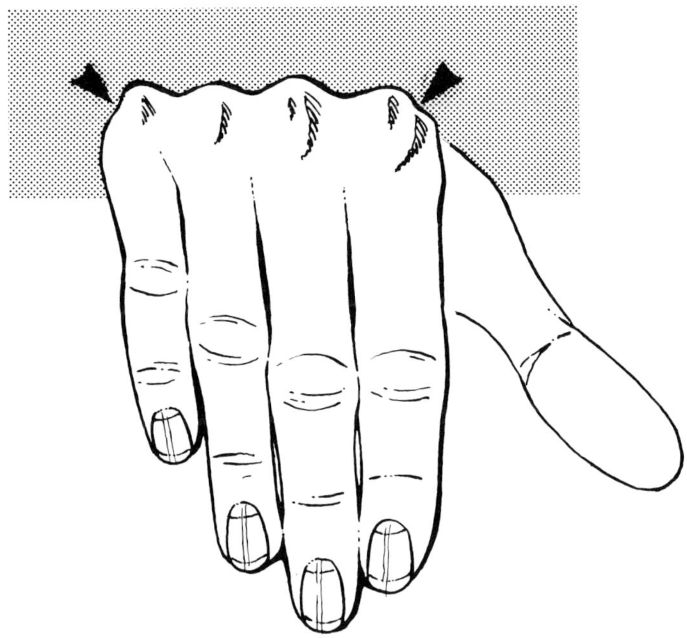

The edge of the proximal phalanx can be felt at the sides of the MCP joint normally

Abnormal

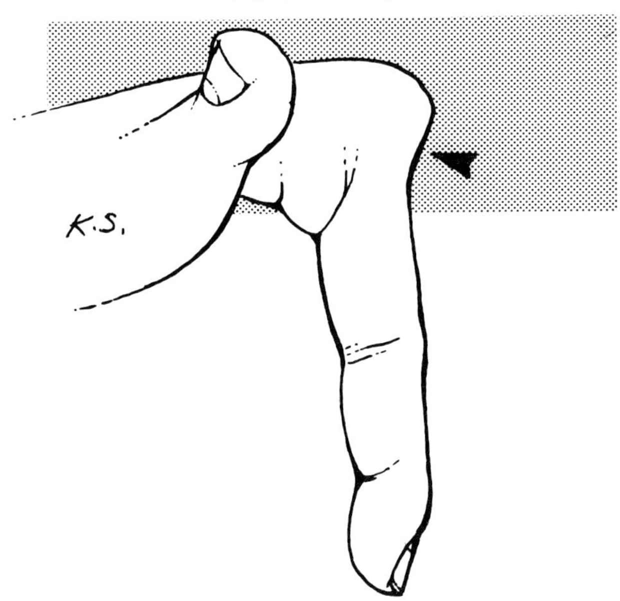

Posterior translocation of the proximal phalanx causes an abnormal "step."

54—Capsular Distension of an IP Joint

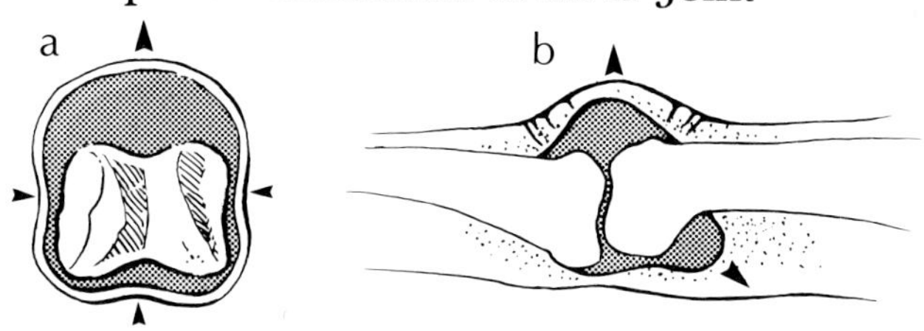

a-The capsule distends when compressed at the sides and bottom

b-The capsule distends when the joint is actively or passively flexed.

Diagram 54. Capsular distension of an IP joint.

Painful areas should be palpated to define the extent of the tenderness. Is the tenderness confined to the articular margins or does it involve the whole joint capsule? Is the tenderness localized to a flexor tendon nodule or is the whole sheath involved? Marked crepitus from joint or tendon sheath may be noted during active assisted movements but the mild crepitus from tenosynovitis may be recognizable only by direct palpation during active movement.

The astute observer will note the temperature of the hand, the presence or absence of sweating, the presence of inappropriate muscle spasm and the presence or absence of callus.

12

The Pelvic Girdle

Donald McGillivray

DEVELOPMENT

The lower limb bud arises opposite the lumbar and upper sacral segments during the 4th week of embryonic life. The ilial cartilages migrate caudally to take a position posterolateral to the coalescing sacral vertebrae. By the tenth week the diarthrodial sacroiliac joint begins to form.

The sacroiliac joint incorporates several sacral segments. The second sacral segment (S2) is always, S1 and S3 usually and L5, L4, and S4 are occasionally incorporated. The sacroiliac joint of the female pelvis usually incorporates fewer segments than the male. At puberty, other gender differences in the shape of the pelvis become apparent. The male pelvis has a narrow funnel shape with strong ligamentous supports. The female pelvis is broader and shorter with less strong ligamentous supports. These differences facilitate parturition.

THE RHEUMATOLOGICAL PHYSICAL EXAMINATION
ISBN 0-8089-1824-9

55— The Post Pubertal Pelvis

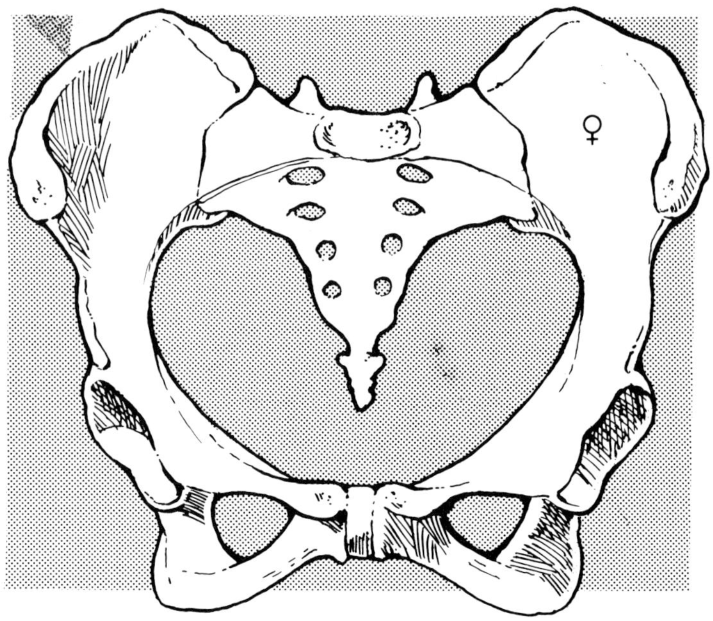

female-shaped like a broad shallow bowl.

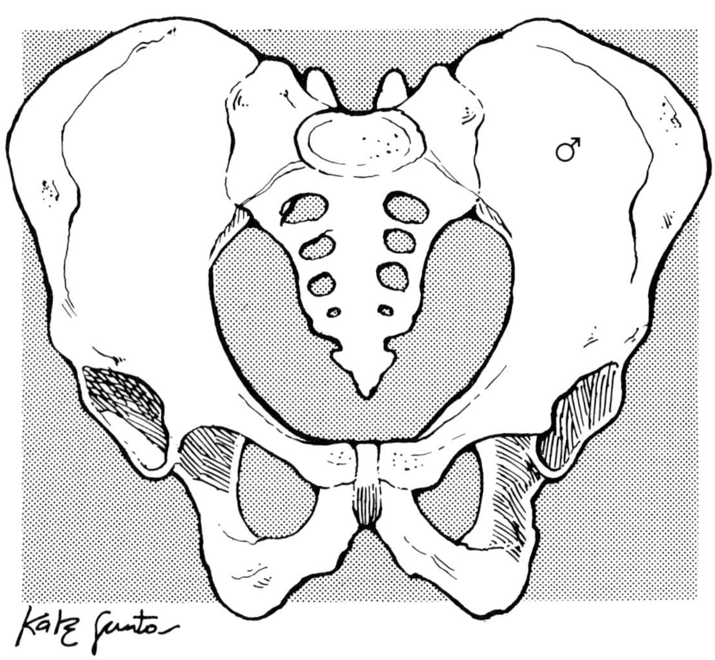

male-shaped like a deep narrow bowl.

Diagram 55. The post pubertal pelvis.

FUNCTIONAL ANATOMY

The solid pelvic girdle transmits the locomotor thrust of the lower limbs to the trunk. In the standing position the pelvic girdle functions like an arch with a reinforcing cross beam.

Bones and Joints

The two irregularly shaped innominate bones join anteriorly at the symphysis pubis. The pubic symphysis has a small articular surface and the ligamentous support is much less than that of the sacroiliac joint. The symphysis is a fibrocartilagenous joint but it may have a central, hyaline lined cleft. The capsule of the symphysis is tight with fibres that are perpendicular to the joint and are arranged circumferentially.

Diagram 56. The sacroiliac joint.

Posteriorly, the sacrum is interposed between the two iliac portions of the innominate bone. The sacroiliac joint has two parts. The anterior part is diarthrodial. The shape and surface of the synovial joint is like an external ear (auricular), facing backwards. Posterior to the auricular portion is the fibrous joint in which the posterior sacroiliac ligament joins the large irregular surfaces of the sacral and iliac tuberosities.

Ligaments

The ligamentous supports of the symphysis pubis are reinforcements of the capsule. There are anterior and posterior sacroiliac ligaments that strengthen the joint and resist rotatory forces.

MOVEMENTS

There is little movement at the sacroiliac joint in the adult. Some flexion/extension of the sacrum can occur. This increases the dimensions of the birth canal and is important in parturition.

PHYSICAL EXAMINATION

Inspection at Rest

The pelvic girdle is not visible due to the thick covering of muscle and fat. In a thin person, the iliac crests and the upper sacral spinous processes can be identified. With the patient standing, observe whether the anterior superior iliac spines are level. The dimples overlying the posterior superior iliac spines should be level also. Abnormalities of shape and size are best studied radiographically.

Inspection with Movement

The movements at the symphysis and the sacroiliac joints are too small to be appreciated clinically. Pain from the pelvic girdle may limit movement of the hip or back.

56— The Sacroiliac Joint

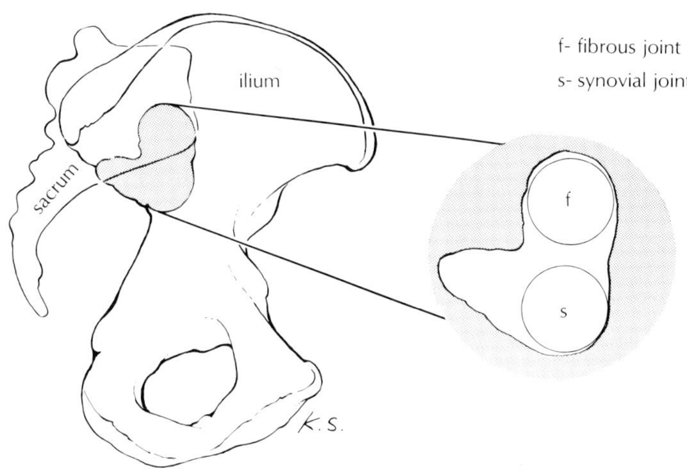

57— Test of Sacroiliac Stress Pain

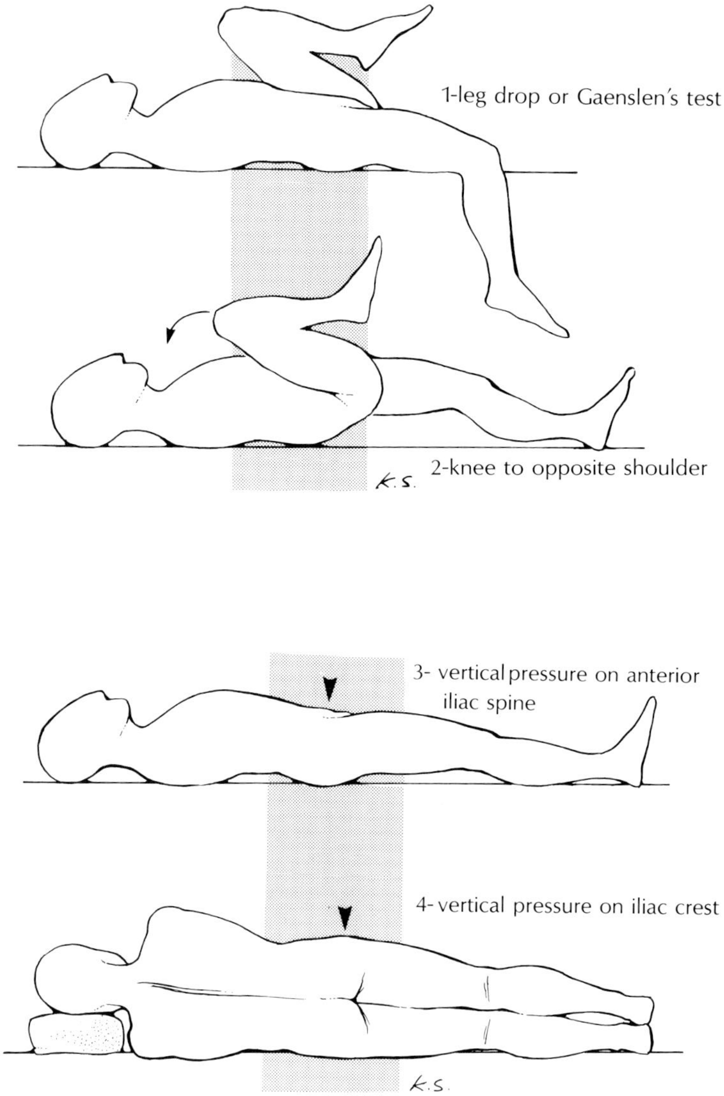

Palpation

With the patient supine the anterior superior iliac spine and the iliac crests are palpated. In the midline, beneath the pubic hair, the fatty mons pubis ("Mountain of Venus") makes the margins of the symphysis indistinct so that only marked swelling or disruption can be recognized. Pressure on a pubic bone may cause differential motion and pain if the joint is unstable.

With the patient in the lateral recumbent position the posterior superior iliac spine can be located beneath the dimple above the buttock. With the hips flexed, the ischial tuberosities can be palpated and then the coccyx is located by palpation in the anal crease posterior to the anus.

The synovial (auricular) part of the sacroiliac joint is too deep to be palpated directly. If the joint is inflamed, there may be tenderness in the soft tissues just below the posterior iliac spine.

Diagram 57. Tests of sacroiliac stress pain.

Indirect Tests for the Pelvic Joints

The pelvic joints cannot be moved directly. The indirect tests, described below, are neither sensitive nor specific. All of these tests stress the sacroiliac joint and produce pain in the buttock. The tests that stress the pelvis using the leg as a lever can be interpreted only if the hip and lower back have been found to be normal.

Gaenslen's Test

With the patient supine, draw one knee up to the chest and lower the other off the examining couch to hyperextend the hip. This will produce pain in the ipsilateral sacroiliac joint if it is inflammed. The same manoeuvre can be done in the lateral recumbent position (Mennell's Test).

Knee-Shoulder Test

The patient is recumbent. One leg is flexed and adducted as far as possible. The examiner then presses the flexed knee firmly toward the opposite shoulder to cause ipsilateral sacroiliac pain.

Compression-Distraction Manoeuvres

These should be done on a firm examining couch. In the recumbent position, both iliac crests are distracted. In the lateral recumbent position, the superior iliac crest is pressed forcibly downward. In the prone position, the lower sacrum is pushed down. These manoeuvres stress both sacroiliac joints.

13

The Hip

Frances Y-K Leung

DEVELOPMENT

Three bones make up the acetabulum but they have one Y-shaped growth plate. Three growth zones produce the eventual shape of the femoral head.

The tri-radiate or Y-shaped cartilage persists as a growth zone between the developing ilium, ischium, and pubis until those bones fuse to form the innominate bone at 20–25 years of age. A rim of cartilage persists around the margin of the acetabulum as the labrum. The acetabulum molds itself around the femoral head.

The upper femur develops from three growth zones. The capital epiphyseal plate is horizontal during most of development, contributing to femoral length. The greater trochanter develops as a traction epiphysis. A growth zone on the superolateral aspect of the femoral neck (femoral neck isthmus) connects these two growth plates and contributes to the width of the femoral neck. Abnormal growth in any of these zones results in abnormally shaped femoral head and reciprocal changes in the acetabulum.

Diagram 58. Growth zones of the hip.

58—Growth Zones of the Hip

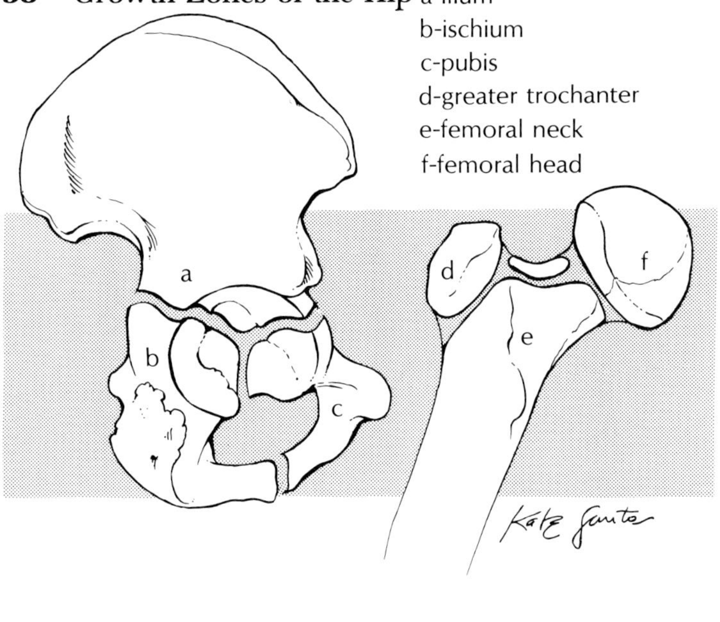

THE RHEUMATOLOGICAL PHYSICAL EXAMINATION
ISBN 0-8089-1824-9

The hip of the embryo is in the flexed, externally rotated position. Initially, the knee points laterally and the sole faces the trunk. By the 7th week of embryonic life, a 90 degree torsion occurs so that the knees point cranially and the soles face caudally. Fetal and postnatal growth includes internal rotation and extension to achieve the normal sagittal alignment by 3 years. Inadequate or excessive rotation leads to toe-out or toe-in deformity.

DEVELOPMENTAL ABNORMALITIES

1. Epiphyseal dysplasia
2. Congenital dislocation of the hip
3. Developmental torsional deformity
4. Protrusio acetabuli (Otto Pelvis)
5. Slipped upper femoral epiphysis

FUNCTIONAL ANATOMY

The Bones and Joints

The acetabulum faces downward, laterally and forward. The femoral neck is directed upward, inward and forward. The flexed, abducted and externally rotated hip of the fetus is fully covered by the acetabulum but in the normal, adult standing position the femoral head is partially uncovered anteriorly.

The rounded femoral head is covered with articular cartilage except where it is joined to the neck and at the attachment of the ligamentum teres (on the opposite pole from the neck). The acetabular surface has a horseshoe shaped articular cartilage, leaving a depressed acetabular notch (like a deep thumb print) to accomodate the ligamentum teres.

59—The Capsule and Ligaments of the Hip

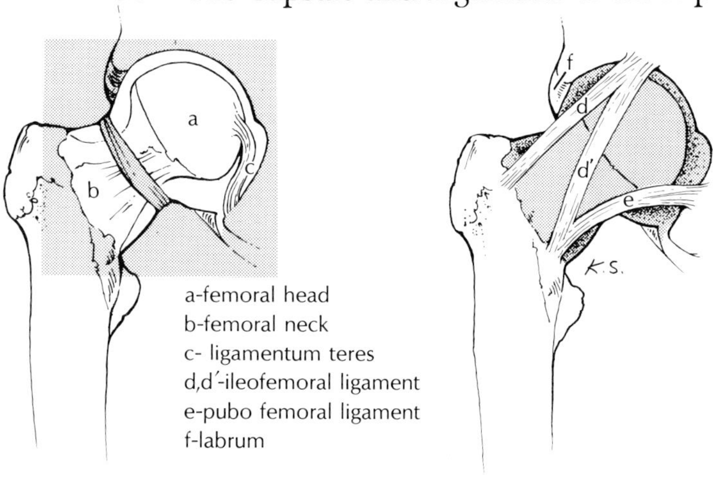

The Capsule and Ligaments

The acetabular labrum increases the depth and size of the cavity so that it is greater than a hemisphere. The capsule extends from the labrum to the neck of the femur enclosing the anterior femoral neck and the upper femur to the intertrochanteric line. Posteriorly, it encloses about half of the femoral neck.

The capsule is strengthened anteriorly by the "Y-shaped" ilio-femoral ligament that prevents excessive extension and stabilizes the hip in the standing position. The pubo-femoral and ischio-femoral ligaments restrict rotation and extension and become slack in the flexed position. A circumferential band of fibrous tissue keeps the capsule snug around the femoral neck.

Diagram 59. The capsule and ligaments of the hip.

A central ligament (ligamentum teres) joins the femoral head to the inferomedial side of the acetabulum. This ligament carries some of the blood supply to the femoral head but contributes little to the stability of the joint.

The hip is very stable. It is virtually impossible to dislocate a normal hip in an adult. In the infant, excessive anteversion or a valgus deformity of the neck make the hip less stable.

Muscles

The muscles around the hip have complex actions. The following list will mention only the main muscles producing the movement described. A more detailed description can be obtained in anatomy or biomechanical texts.

Flexors	iliopsoas, pectineus, (rectus femoris)
Extensors	gluteus maximus and adductor magnus, (hamstrings)
Abductors	gluteus medius and minimus,
Adductors	adductor magnus, brevis, longus and gracilis
Rotators	
medial	gluteus medius and minimus, anterior fibres tensor fasciae latae
lateral	piriformis, obturator, gemelli
	gluteus medius and minimus, posterior fibres

MOVEMENTS

The hip is a ball and socket joint that allows the thigh great freedom of movement. The range of movement is influenced by the position of the low back, the knee, and the opposite hip. Flexion of the hip is increased if the knee and the low back are also flexed. Extension of the hip is increased if the knee is extended. Abduction is increased if both hips are slightly flexed.

PHYSICAL EXAMINATION OF THE HIP

Inspection at Rest

The hip joint is difficult to examine. It is too deep to observe directly so that its position has to be deduced by careful observation of the surface anatomy of the pelvis. Too often, this fundamental information is obscured due to excessive modesty on the part of the patient or embarrassment on the part of the examiner. Unless the pelvis can be observed satisfactorily, the hip cannot be examined properly.

Diagram 60. Flexion and rotational deformity of the hip.

A flexion deformity of the hip can be hidden by hyperextension of the spine. A marked lumbar lordosis should alert the examiner to the possibility of a flexion deformity of the hip. Adduction or abduction deformities can be masked by tilting the pelvis and compensating in the lumbar spine. The patient should be inspected in the standing position to ensure that the spine is straight and the iliac crests are level.

Rotational deformities are observed best from the front with the patient standing. A vertical line from the mid-point of the inguinal ligament should cross the middle of the patella and the middle of the ankle. Rotational deformities are recognized as deviations from this alignment.

Lengthening or shortening cannot be differentiated from an angulation deformity by simple inspection. Leg length must be measured.

60— Flexion Deformity of the Hip

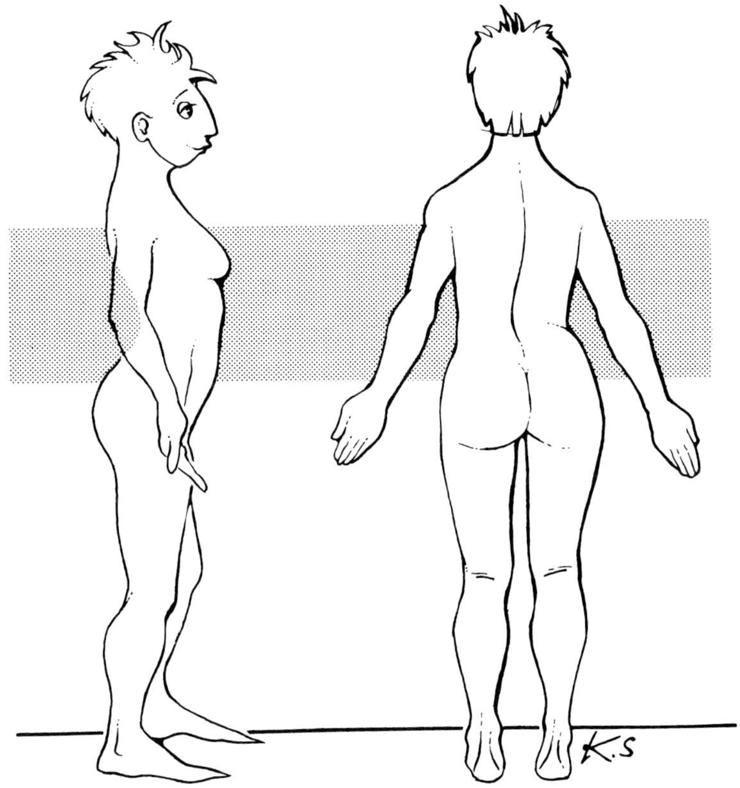

Note excessive lumbar lordosis and slight flexion of the knee to achieve an erect stance.

60— Rotational Deformity of the Hip

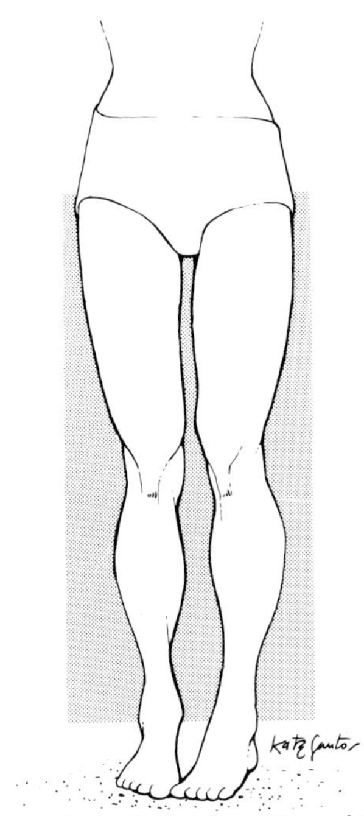

Note internal rotation of the left thigh and leg due to excessive anteversion of the hip.

61—Measurement Technique for Leg Length

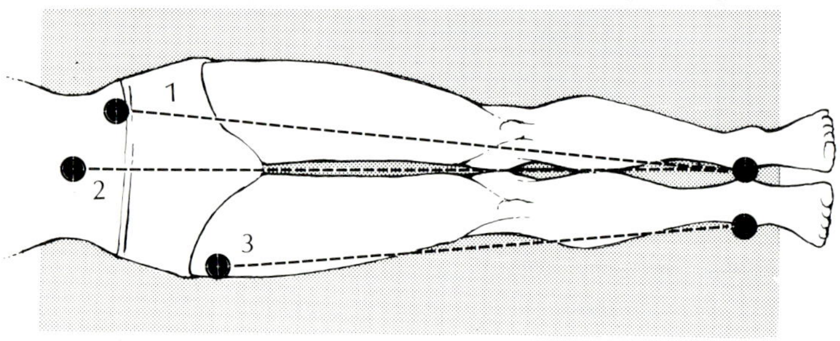

1-true leg length
2-apparent leg length
3-trochanter to malleolar length,to determine if shortening is in femoral neck or above.

62—Trendelenburg Test

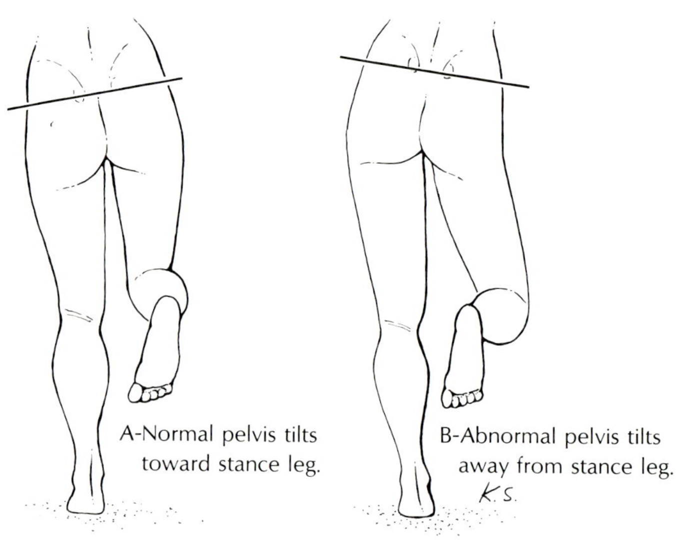

Diagram 61. Measurement technique for leg length.

If a difference is noted, the examiner then measures from the greater trochanter to the medial malleolus to determine whether the shortening is below the femoral neck or above. A number of clinical measurements have been proposed to assess shortening of the femoral neck or head, but the clinical measures are much less accurate than radiological studies.

Special Tests

Trendelenburg Test

The patient stands on one leg. The examiner, standing or seated behind the patient, supports the trunk in the erect position and notes whether the pelvis rises or falls on the non-stance side. Normally, the abductors will pull the pelvis over the hip, raising the non-stance side. If the muscles are weak or if the hip is subluxed or dislocated so that the muscles cannot shorten adequately, then the pelvis will fall on the non-stance side producing a positive test.

Diagram 62. Trendelenburg Test.

The common causes of a positive Trendelenburg test are; hip disease, an L5 nerve root lesion and conditions characterized by generalized muscle weakness. In the first two situations the abnormality is usually unilateral and in the latter it is bilateral.

Thomas Test

A flexion deformity of the hip is measured by bringing both knees to the chest until the lumbar spine is flat then each leg is lowered in turn to the limit of extension. The presence of a flexion deformity is demonstrated by the inability to rest the leg on the couch. The remaining angle is recorded as a flexion deformity and the range is expressed as the abnormal position to the fully flexed position, e.g. hip flexion, right 20 degrees to 100 degrees, left 0 degrees to 120 degrees (normal).

14

The Knee

Arthur Bookman

DEVELOPMENT

At 6 weeks of embryonic life, the lower limb bud develops a central expansion where flexion occurs to become the knee. By the 7th–8th week the lower limb rotates medially so that the knee points toward the head and the axis of movement swings toward the sagittal plane.

Diagram 63. The developing limb bud.

63— The Developing Limb Bud

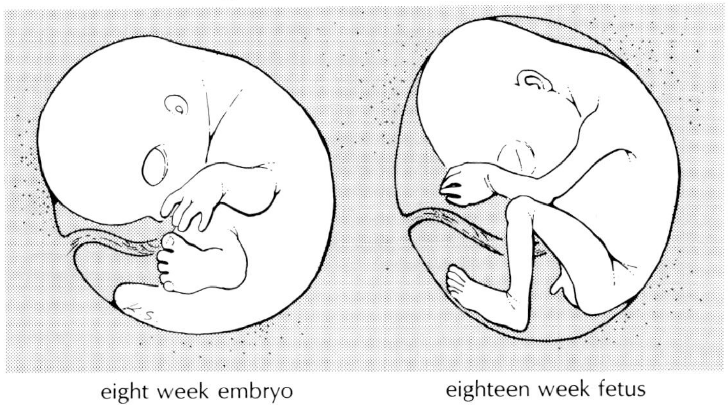

THE RHEUMATOLOGICAL PHYSICAL EXAMINATION
ISBN 0-8089-1824-9

67—The Menisci

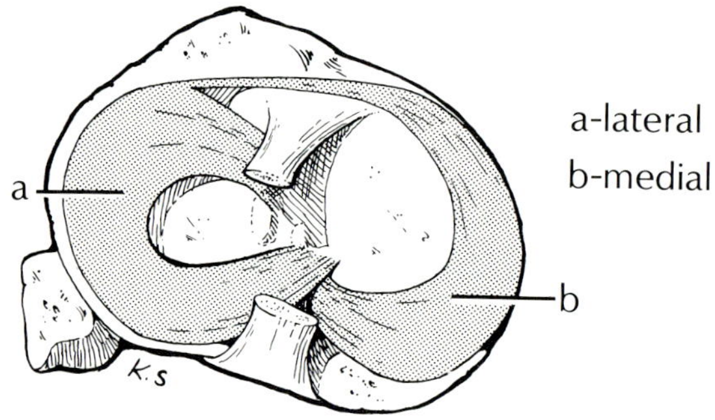

tibial plateau,seen from above to show the menisci

68—Collateral Ligaments from the Lateral Aspect

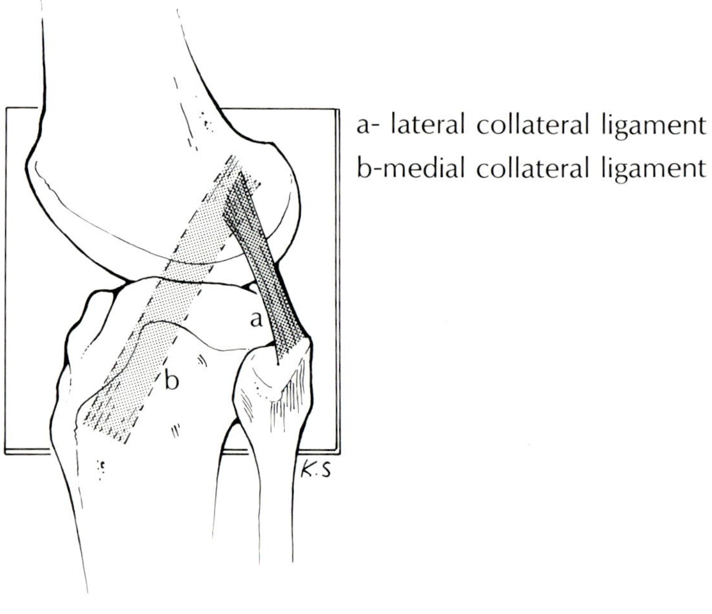

Diagram 67. To show menisci.

The menisci have concave superior surfaces to accommodate the femur, as it rotates. The inferior sufaces are flattened to allow them to slide forward and back with the femur over the tibia. The menisci are attached centrally to the tibial intercondylar tubercles. The circumference of the medial meniscus is firmly attached to the surrounding structures. The lateral meniscus is loosely attached to the capsule around its circumference and is much more mobile.

The Ligaments

The collateral ligaments become taut in extension, stabilizing the knee in the coronal plane and preventing external rotation of the tibia on the femur.

Diagram 68. The collateral ligaments.

The cruciate ligaments stabilize the knee in the sagittal plane and prevent internal rotation of the tibia when the knee is extended. The cruciates are named according to their tibial attachments. The anterior cruciate is directed upward, backward, and laterally. The posterior cruciate is directed upward, forward, and medially. They are attached in front of and behind the intercondylar tubercles of the tibia and to the inner surface of the femoral condyles. The cruciates are partly covered by synovial tissue and thus can be considered to be reinforcements of the capsule.

During flexion, the anterior cruciate prevents the femur from rolling backward off the tibia, forcing it to slide as it rolls. The posterior cruciate prevents the femur from rolling off the front of the tibia during extension. The cruciates become coiled and taut in internal rotation, preventing this movement when the knee is extended.

Diagram 69. The cruciate ligaments.

The posterior capsule is very strong, reinforced by capsular bands and muscles. This limits extension of the knee. Flexion is limited by impingement of the calf and thigh muscles when the hip is flexed. When the hip is extended, flexion is limited by tension in the quadriceps mechanism.

Muscles

The extensor muscle of the knee is the quadriceps (4 heads; the rectus and 3 vasti). The rectus femoris originates from the anterior superior iliac spine and inserts through the patellar tendon to the tibial tuberosity. It acts as a hip flexor and knee extensor. The vasti arise from the front and sides of the femur and insert with the rectus. The vastus medialis is particularly active in the last few degrees of extension taking part in the locking or "screw home" medial rotation of the femur on the tibia.

The main flexor muscles are the hamstrings. These are the semimembranosus and semitendinosus on the medial side and the biceps femoris on the lateral side. Ancillary flexors are the gracilis, sartorius, and medial gastrocnemius on the medial side and the popliteus and lateral gastrocnemius on the lateral side. The hamstrings are more effective if the hip is flexed.

69—Cruciate Ligaments Seen from the Lateral Side

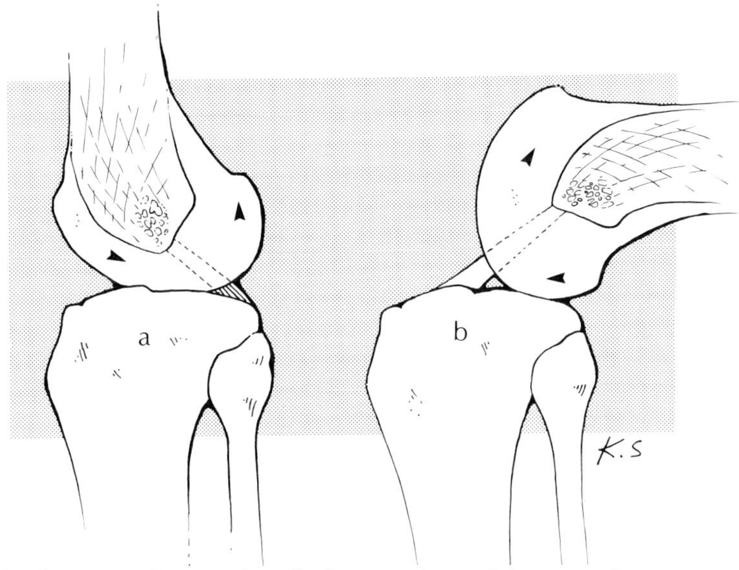

a-the posterior cruciate limits anterior roll in extension
b-the anterior cruciate limits posterior roll in flexion.

69—Cruciate Ligaments Seen from Above

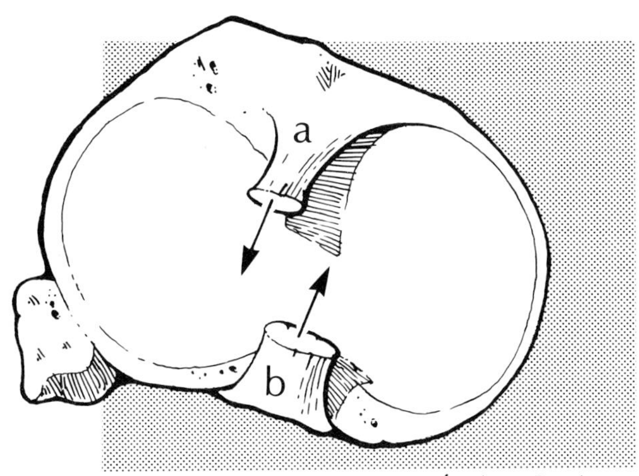

a-anterior cruciate
b-posterior cruciate

70—Normal Alignment of the Knee

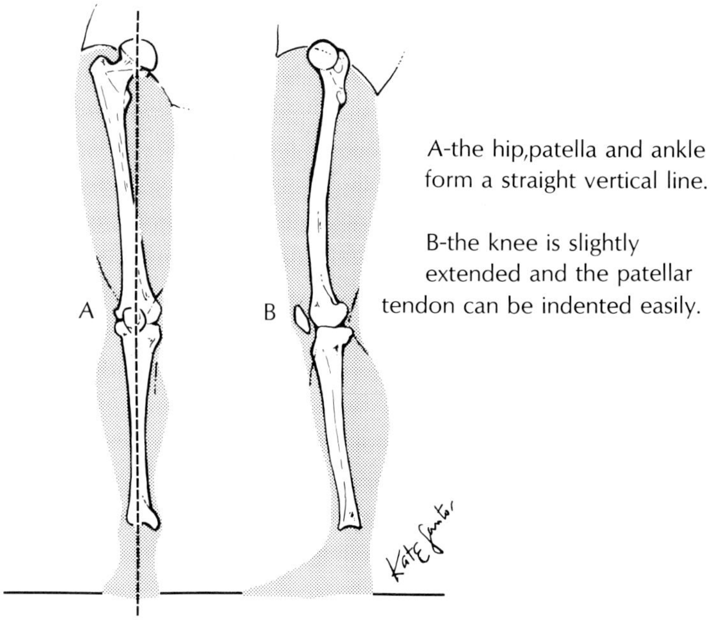

71—The Knee, Sagittal Alignment

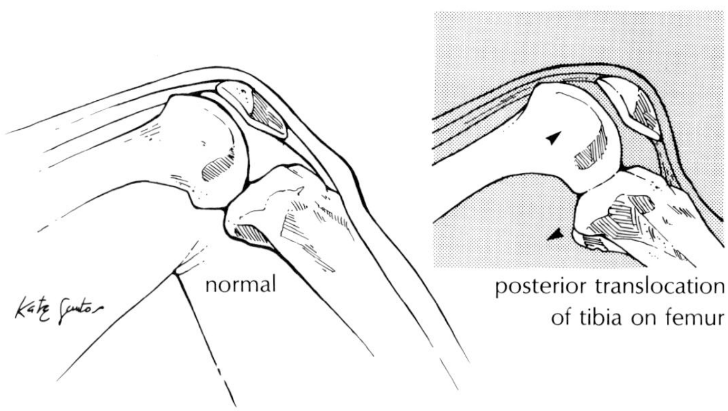

The lateral hamstrings and the tensor fascia lata externally rotate the tibia. The medial hamstrings and the popliteus internally rotate the tibia. When standing, the foot and tibia are fixed and the rotator muscles move the body and thigh on the leg.

Movement

The knee hinges from full extension to a maximal flexion of 160 degrees. When the knee is flexed, the tibia can rotate on the femur, 30 degrees internally and 40 degrees externally.

PHYSICAL EXAMINATION

The knee should be inspected with the patient standing, walking, sitting, and recumbent. Malalignment may become apparent only in the standing position and a popliteal (Baker's) cyst is most prominent with the patient standing. Abnormalities of movement may be evident only when the patient walks or climbs.

Inspection at Rest

In the coronal plane, angulation can be recognized when a line from the middle of the inguinal ligament to the mid point of the ankle fails to cross the centre of the patella. Medial angulation at the knee is known as genu varus, lateral angulation as genu valgus.

In the normal upright stance, the patellar tendon is relaxed and the knee is slightly extended. Angular deformities in the sagittal plane include flexion deformity and hyperextension (genu recurvatum).

Diagram 70. Alignment of the knee.

Translocations are difficult to identify by inspection. With the patient supine and the knee bent to 90 degrees, one can see that the point of angulation occurs at the upper pole of the patella. The patella and the patellar tendon are in line with the anterior tibial border. In this position, posterior translocation is noted when the proximal tibia sags posteriorly.

Diagram 71. Posterior translocation of tibia.

Frontal inspection with the patient seated will reveal rotation deformities. Rotation may occur through the joint causing a deviation of the patella and patellar tendon. Deviation may occur in the tibia (tibial torsion), leaving the patella and patellar tendon in normal alignment.

Collapse of bone and cartilage in one tibiofemoral compartment leads to an angular deformity. Collapse of both tibiofemoral compartments leads to a loss of length.

Intra capsular swelling of the knee can be recognized when the suprapatellar pouch is distended. This is most obvious when the knee is extended. With flexion, the posterior capsule of the knee is relaxed and fluid can be accomodated at the back.

Diagram 72. Synovial pouches.

There are more than 11 bursae around the knee. Three of these communicate with the joint (the suprapatellar, the popliteus, and the medial gastrocnemius) and may become visibily distended when there is a knee effusion. Inflamed bursae can produce localized swellings around the knee.

Diagram 73. Knee bursae.

Bony enlargement of the articular margins can cause visible deformity. Large medial fat pads can distort the appearance of the knee. These seldom occur without similar fatty deposits around the thighs and buttocks. Muscular wasting should be noted.

Inspection with Movement

Figure 23. Hip and knee flexion.

The patient is asked to stand with the knees fully extended and then, when practical, to perform a full squat. If difficulties are encountered, the patient is asked to lie supine and actively flex and extend the knee. The examiner watches for restriction, guarding, or interrupted movement.

72—Synovial Pouches in Extension and Flexion

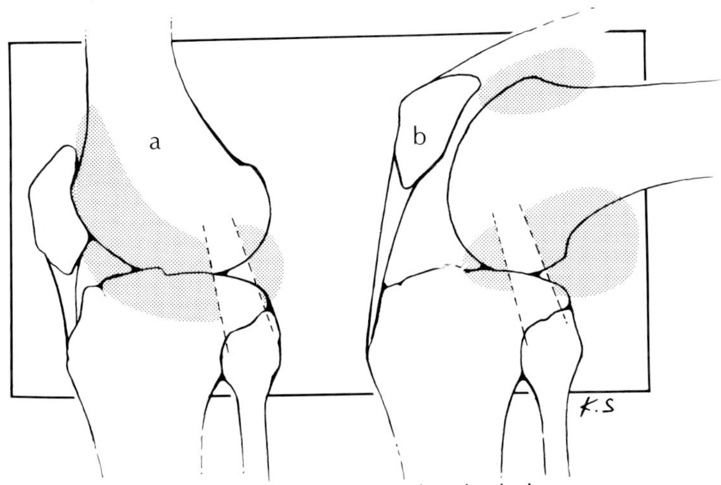

The synovial pouches are shown by the shaded areas.
In extension a-the posterior capsule is taut forcing fluid forward.
In flexion b-fluid fluid can be accomodated posteriorly.

73—Bursae around the Knee

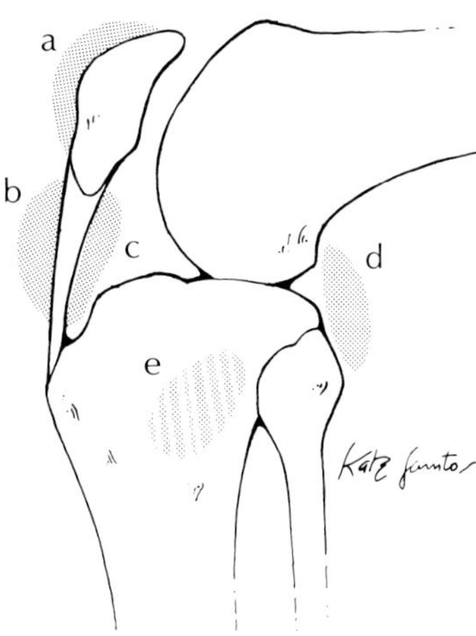

a-prepatellar bursae
b-infrapatellar bursa
c-subpatellar bursa
d-semimembranosus bursa
e-anserine bursa on the medial side of the knee.

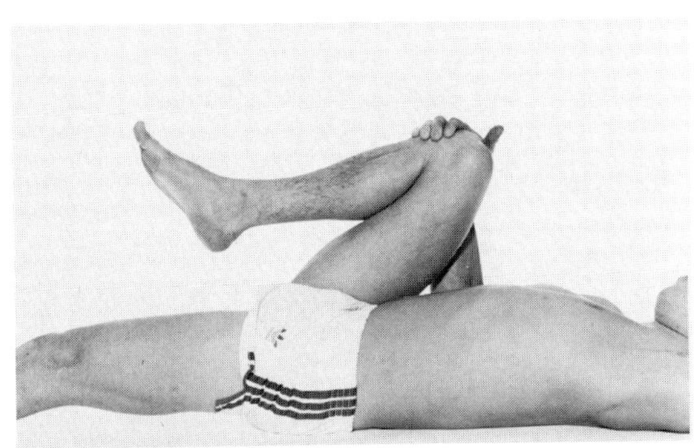

Figure 23

74—Rotation of the Tibia

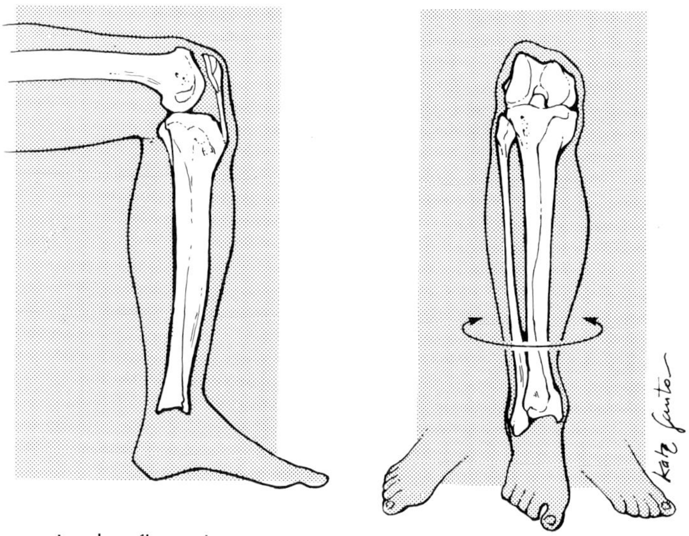

In the flexed position the collateral and cruciate ligaments are relaxed allowing rotation of the tibia on the femur.

Palpation

Active Assisted and Passive Movement

The patient, lying supine, actively extends the knee. If there is restriction, the examiner assists extension by lifting the heel. This will correct an extension lag but not a flexion contracture. A lag of more than 5 degrees is abnormal. Assisted and passive movement can quantitate the degree of restriction and assess the quality of the end point. Forced flexion and extension will reveal stress pain in an inflamed knee.

Diagnostic Palpation

With the knee in 90 degrees of flexion, most of the the joint margin can be palpated. It is obscured anteriorly by the patellar tendon, laterally by the collateral ligaments and posteriorly by the muscles and the neurovascular bundle. The anterior surface of the femoral condyles are palpable. Note that the anterior edge of the tibial plateau protrudes slightly in front of the femoral condyles. The protrusion is more marked on the lateral side. Translocation of the knee, in the sagittal plane, alters this normal relationship.

Swelling at the knee is palpated to determine its boundaries, depth, and consistency. Effusions in the knee are demonstrated by the bulge sign and balloon sign (illustrated in Chapter 3). The patient is supine and the knee is extended. The bulge sign is produced by moving the fluid from one recess up into the suprapatellar pouch. Then the stroke is reversed, moving the fluid back into the recess resulting in a sudden bulge. This manoeuvre demonstrates small effusions but a large effusion is not demonstrable.

To perform the balloon sign the examiner compresses the suprapatellar pouch with one hand while palpating the lateral recesses with the other. Pressure in one area causes distension of the other. The balloon sign is used for large effusions.

The "patellar tap" is a modification of the balloon sign that requires enough intra-articular fluid to lift the patella off the femur. The examiner presses sharply on the patella. As the patella descends, it displaces the fluid to the lateral recesses and the suprapatellar pouch. Then it hits the front of the femur with an easily palpable bump. When the pressure is released, it rises so that the manoeuvre can be repeated. This is an impressive sign but it is often absent despite large effusions. If the knee isn't fully extended or if the quadriceps isn't relaxed, the tension in the extensor apparatus will hold the patella firmly on the femur, precluding a "tap". A large subpatellar fat pad may give a false positive "tap". This test is less sensitive and no more specific than the balloon sign.

Both ends of the patellar tendon and the subpatellar fat pad should be examined and the collateral ligaments should be palpated throughout their course. Angular deformities are measured with a goniometer. Rotational deformities are measured by rotating the tibia on the femur with the knee flexed to 90 degrees. The tibia should rotate 30 degrees internally and 40 degrees externally. The resting position and the range of rotation should be recorded. Note that there is no rotation in the extended position in a normal knee.

Diagram 74. Rotation of the tibia.

Effusions may become loculated in synovial cysts in the popliteal fossa (Baker's Cyst). These cysts communicate with the knee. Forced flexion of the knee may raise the pressure in the joint and the cyst so that the latter ruptures into the calf causing pain, swelling and a characteristic crescent shaped bruise in the calf, (crescent sign). These cysts are palpable at the posterior aspect of the knee and upper calf with the knee slightly bent. Sometimes a small cyst is easier to feel with the patient lying prone.

Diagram 75. The collateral stress test.

The collateral ligaments are tested by applying selective stress. The medial collateral is tested by applying force to the outside of the knee and a counter force to the inside of the ankle and the reverse position is used to test the lateral ligament. With the knee fully extended, the collateral ligaments are tight and no movement is possible in a normal knee. With slight flexion a bit of rocking is possible in the normal knee but this is painless and the end point is firm.

The cruciate ligaments prevent anterior/posterior instability and limit medial rotation. With the knee flexed to 90 degrees and the leg hanging, the upper tibia is pulled forward to test the anterior cruciate and pushed backward to test the posterior cruciate (Drawer sign). The examiner should sit, facing the knee, both hands grasping the upper tibia and the index fingers should indent the hamstring tendons to ensure that the muscles are relaxed.

Diagram 76. The drawer sign.

If the hamstrings are contracted, the tibia cannot be drawn forward and an anterior cruciate injury may be missed. If the posterior cruciate is torn and the hamstrings have drawn the tibia as far back as the collateral ligaments will allow, a pull will result in great anterior movement simulating an anterior cruciate tear. The hamstrings must be relaxed and the tibia positioned normally relative to the femur before the Drawer sign is attempted.

The tibia should be rotated by grasping and twisting the foot while stabilizing the femur with the other hand. Internal rotation of more than 30 degrees suggests a cruciate injury. External rotation of more than 40 degrees suggests a collateral injury.

75— Collateral Stress Test

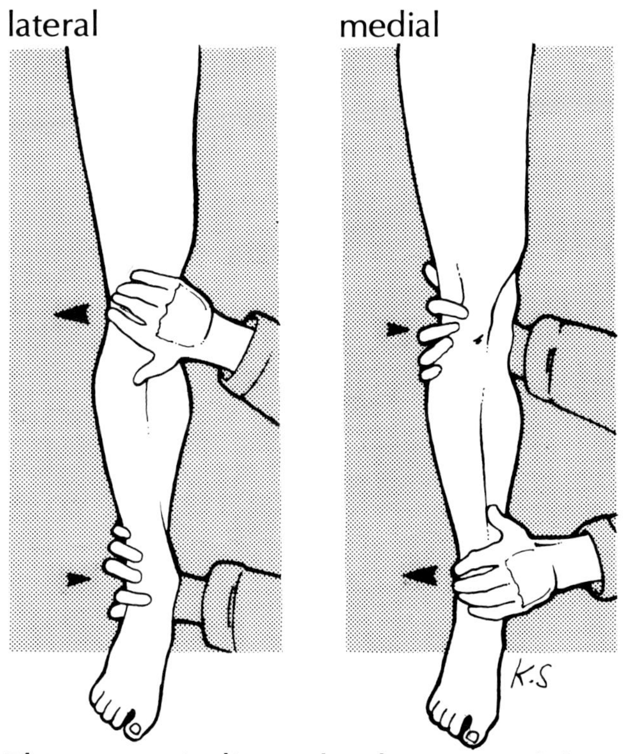

The arrows indicate the direction of the stress.

76— Drawer Sign—Cruciate Stress Test

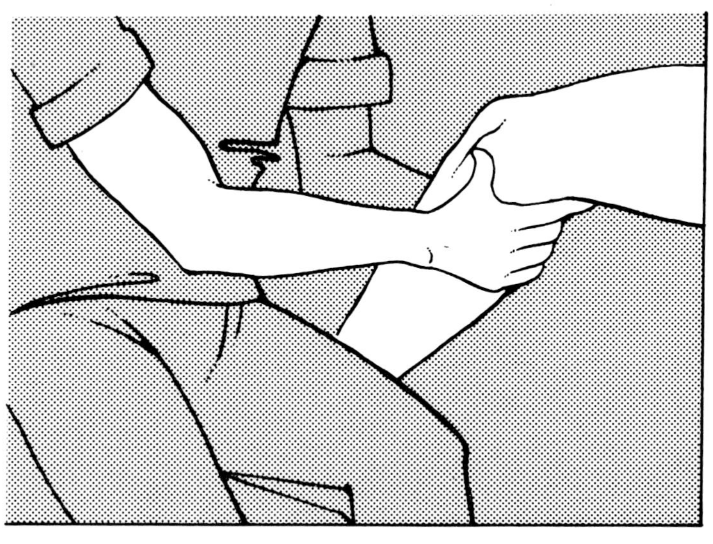

Patellofemoral instability is assessed by moving the patella from side to side with the knee extended and the quadriceps relaxed. A small amount of movement is normal. A patient with recurrent subluxation of the patella may resist or express apprehension as the patella is moved laterally (patellar apprehension test).

The quality of the patellofemoral cartilage can be assessed by palpating over the patella during active movement. Pressure on the patella may cause pain at the same time as crepitus is felt, suggesting severe degeneration.

Special Tests

There are many tests, with many variations, that are used to detect damage to menisci and ligaments. Although these tests are the province of the orthopedist, the rheumatologist should become familiar with them if the pattern of practice warrants. The classic tests are described below and further details are available through the references in the reading list.

Meniscal Injuries

A torn meniscus may cause joint line tenderness without bony enlargement. Occasionally, a meniscal tear will result in a tag that can catch between the articular surfaces and prevent movement. Since the posterior horns are compressed in full flexion and the anterior horns in full extension, noting the degree of flexion helps to localize a lesion.

McMurray's Test. The patient is recumbent, with the knee and hip fully flexed and the heel is grasped by the examiner's hand. The examiner palpates the joint margin with the fingers and thumb of the other hand. The knee is then gradually extended passively with a valgus stress and maximal internal rotation and then maximal external rotation. While performing the test, the examiner feels and listens for a click and notes the degree of flexion when this occurs. A painful click, felt at the beginning of extension is suggestive of a torn meniscus.

Apley's Test. The patient is prone with the knee flexed to 90 degrees. The examiner compresses the menisci by pressing down on the foot while rotating, flexing and extending the knee. Normally, this results in a painless smooth movement. A recent meniscal injury will be painful with compression and the torn fragments may produce a click. Distracting the joint by pulling on the tibia and pushing on the thigh will be painless in a pure meniscal injury but painful if a ligament is damaged.

Rotational Instability

Pivot Shift. This test is used to define anterolateral instability. The patient lies supine with the leg extended. The examiner supports the leg and internally rotating the heel with one hand to anteriorly rotate the lateral tibia. Applying a slight valgus stress to the knee with the other hand, the extended knee is slowly flexed. The lateral tibial plateau falls into place with a 'clunk' at about 30 degrees of flexion, producing a positive test. A tear of the anterior cruciate and the lateral collateral ligament will give a pivot shift.

Slocum Test. This test is used to define anteromedial instability. An anterior Drawer sign is not rectified by external rotation of the tibia on the femur. This indicates laxity of the medial collateral as well as the anterior cruciate ligaments.

15

The Ankle and Foot

Adel G. Fam

DEVELOPMENT

The lower limb buds first appear about the 4th week of embryonic life. Each limb bud develops in a proximo-distal sequence. Between the 6th and 8th week, the distal part of the limb bud shows digital segmentation or "toe ray" and the cartilage precursors of future bones become separate.

At birth, the relationship between the foot and leg is normal and the apparent inversion is due to the slight varus angulation of the knee. The bones of the foot are still largely cartilagenous and thus are still deformable. Ossification occurs throughout the first three years. Fusion of the phalangeal and metatarsal epiphyses is complete by late adolescence.

The longitudinal arch usually begins to appear by the third year but may be delayed until early adolescence.

THE RHEUMATOLOGICAL PHYSICAL EXAMINATION
ISBN 0-8089-1824-9

77— Talipes

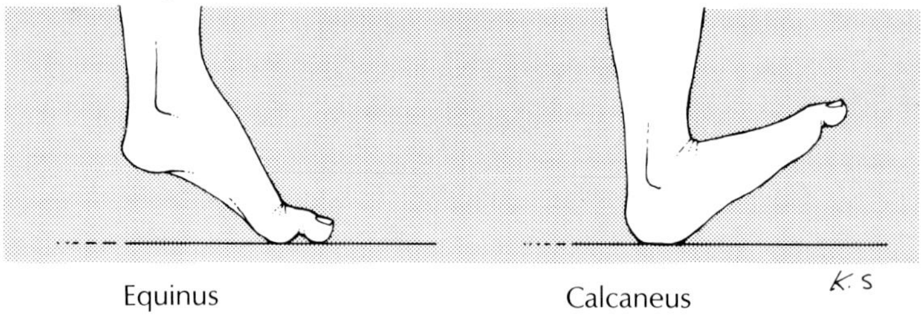

78— Bones of the Foot

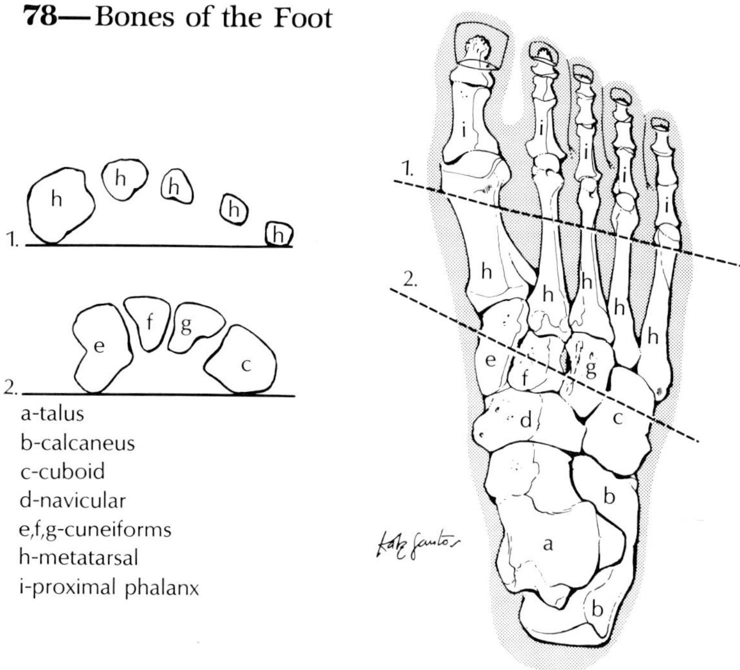

DEVELOPMENTAL ABNORMALITIES

Hindfoot

Talipes or "club foot" refers to a deformity of the ankle and foot (tali=ankle, pes=foot). Equinus (like a horse) is a plantar flexed ankle. Calcaneus is a dorsi flexed ankle. These deformities are often associated with midfoot abnormalities such as talipes equinovarus and talipes calcaneovalgus.

Diagram 77. Clubfoot.

Midfoot

Pes planus or "flat foot" is the absence of a normal longitudinal arch. Pes cavus is a heightened longitudinal arch. These abnormalities are often associated with valgus and varus deformities respectively. Tarsal coalition is characterized by abnormal fibrous, cartilagenous or bony connections between the bones of the hind and midfoot.

Forefoot

All the metatarsals may be adducted, i.e., metatarsus varus. More commonly, only the first ray is adducted, metatarsus primus varus, which may precede a hallux valgus deformity.

Developmental abnormalities of the toes include; adactyly (aplasia or hypoplasia of the digits), hypodactyly (decreased numbers of digits), polydactyly (supernumerary digits), syndactyly (joined digits) and brachydactyly (short digits).

FUNCTIONAL ANATOMY

Bones

The foot has three functional units; the hindfoot, the midfoot and the forefoot. The hindfoot contains the calcaneus and the talus. The midfoot contains the five small tarsal bones and the forefoot contains the metatarsals and phalanges.

Diagram 78. The bones of the foot.

The calcaneus is large and oblong. The anterior ⅔ support and articulate with the talus. The posterior ⅓ forms the prominence of the heel and rests on the ground. The anterior surface articulates with the cuboid. There is a medial projection, the sustentaculum tali, which is joined to the navicular by a strong "spring" ligament.

The talus has a body, neck, and head. The body rests upon the anterior ⅔ of the calcaneus. Its upper surface is dome-shaped with flattened sides. It articulates with the tibia above and the malleoli on the sides. The head is rounded anteriorly and fits into the cupped surface of the navicular. The talus is the link between the leg and the foot with the ankle joint forming the proximal connection to the leg and the subtalar joint forming the distal connection to the foot.

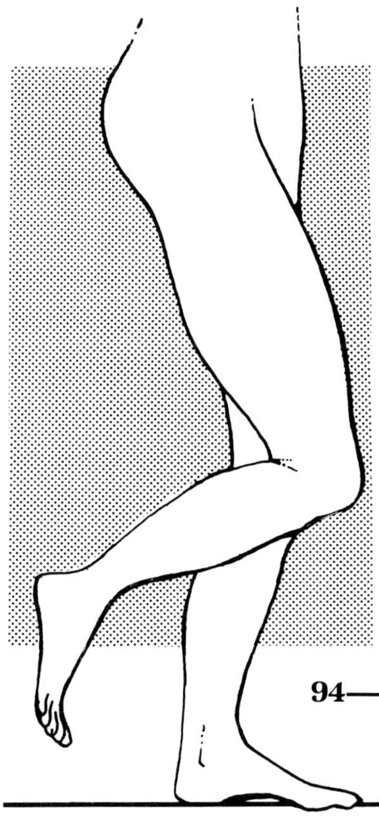

94—

swing/mid-stance

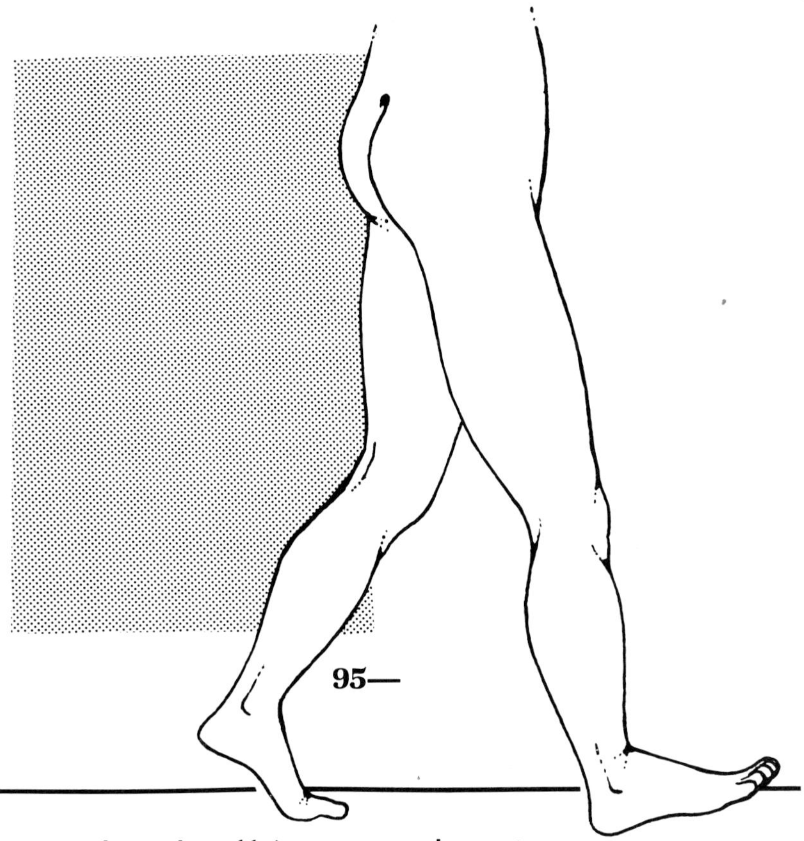

95—

heel off/terminal swing

Diagram 94. Midstance.

Midstance — Acceleration to Mid Swing

The right leg moves over the foot at the ankle joint. The knee flexes slightly and the quadriceps become active to support the weight and limit knee flexion. The right gluteus medius contracts to keep the pelvis level.

After the toe off, the left knee bends to lift the foot clear of the ground and the iliopsoas swings the leg forward.

Diagram 95. Heel off.

Heel Off — Terminal Swing and Heel Strike

The weight moves forward onto the right forefoot. The right heel rises and the great toe dorsi flexes.

The left quadriceps has pulled the knee straight and the tibialis anterior has dorsi flexed the ankle. The forward swing of the left leg is checked by the hamstrings and the gluteus maximus. The left heel strikes the ground.

The process is then repeated with the left leg providing support while the right leg is advanced.

96— Trunk and Arm Movements with Gait

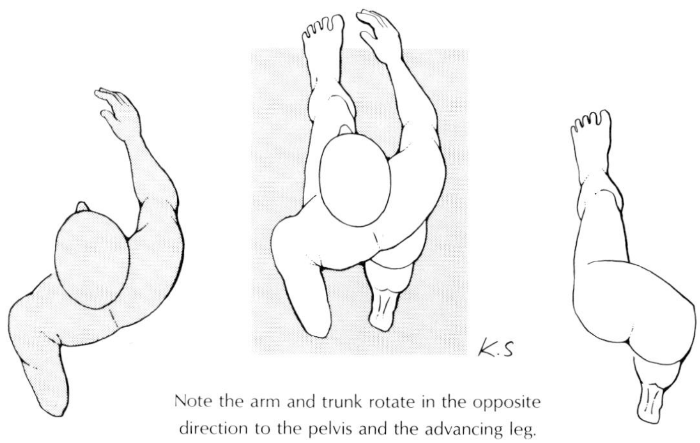

Note the arm and trunk rotate in the opposite direction to the pelvis and the advancing leg.

Diagram 96. Arm and trunk movements.

Arm and Trunk Movements

Continue walking and note that the pelvis advances with the swing leg by rotating on the stance hip. The chest and shoulders do not rotate. The rotation of the pelvis is compensated by derotation in the lower thoracic spine. The arms move with the opposite leg.

Physical Examination of Gait

Observations must be organized, examining each functional segment (foot, ankle, knee, hip, and trunk) in both the stance and swing phase.

Simplified Classification of Gait Disturbance

1. Biomechanical Problems
   Painless, e.g. short femur/tibia genu valgum/varum toe in or toe out
   Painful, e.g. fractures, Inflammatory or degenerative joint disease
2. Neuromuscular Disease
   Weakness, e.g. drop foot, Trendelenberg limp, Muscular Dystrophy
   Imbalance, e.g. Cerebral Palsy, Hemiplegia
   Loss of Sensation, e.g. Diabetes mellitus, Tabes dorsalis
3. Associated Disease, e.g. back pain, hysteria, amputation

Inspection

The patient should be observed while walking for a minimum of several yards. The patient should be disrobed to allow an adequate view of the legs and pelvis. Barefoot is best.

Foot and Ankle. Does the heel strike? Does the foot pronate slightly in mid stance? Does the heel rise before a vigorous push off? Does the ankle dorsi flex normally so that the foot is positioned for the next heel strike?

Knee. Is the knee fully extended at heel strike and does it flex slightly through mid stance. Does the knee flex adequately in the swing phase to allow the foot to swing forward without touching the ground?

Hip. Is the hip flexed at heel strike and extended at toe off? Is the pelvis level and does it rotate forward with the advancing leg?

Patterns of Antalgic Gait

Due to pain, the patient hurries off one leg and spends the greater part of the gait cycle on the other. The site of pain can result in characteristic modifications of the antalgic gait

Painful Forefoot

The forefoot is protected from weight bearing. The heel does not rise in the late stance phase. The knee, hip and trunk bend to maintain forward movement. The swing phase on the pain free side is shortened so that the knee does not fully extend. There is no push off.

This gait can be recognized by forward "bobbing" in the late stance phase on the painful side.

Painful Forefeet

Painful forefeet result in a shuffling gait. There is no push off. The step is short. The hips and knees remain slightly flexed. Body movements are controlled to ensure that the centre of gravity remains well forward so that a push off will not be required.

Painful Midfoot

The foot is held in an inverted (supinated) position and the push off is from the lateral side. This keeps the foot in its most rigid position and lessens midfoot movement.

Painful Heel

There is no heel strike. The foot is placed flat on the floor or the heel may be kept off the floor. The swing phase on the painful side is shortened and the knee doesn't fully extend.

If the pain arises at the achilles tendon insertion, push off is avoided and the gait resembles that of the painful forefoot.

Painful Ankle

The leg may be externally rotated and slightly abducted, similar to the gait produced by a below knee cast. This lessens movement through the ankle.

Painful Knee

A painful effusion results in a slightly flexed knee. The pain prevents full extension at the end of the swing phase and the heel strike is softened. A damaged knee may be held stiffly. The body then pivots around the leg during the stance phase and the leg is swung forward by circumduction. This gait is similiar to that produced by a stove pipe cast.

Painful Hip

There is usually some flexion of the body over the hip. Stance is accompanied by lateral "bobbing" of the body over the painful hip to decrease the pull of the gluteus medius.

Painful Low Back

The low back is flattened and held rigidly. The pelvis does not rotate with the advancing leg but remains aligned with the thorax. This results in a shortened step and considerable caution when turning.

17

Measurement of Muscle Strength

Antoine Helewa

Accurate estimates of muscle strength are important in certain rheumatic diseases, both as a diagnostic and prognostic tool and as a guide for clinicians in evaluating the effects of drug therapy and therapeutic exercises.

The measures most commonly used are the British Medical Research Council (MRC) scale and simple weight lifting techniques. The MRC scale lacks precision and weight lifting techniques require an assortment of weights.

The clinician needs a method that is: (1) quantitative, so that numbers may be produced, (2) objective, so that observer impressions do not affect the measurement values, (3) sensitive to changes in muscle strength, (4) reliable, in that the instrument is free from defect and does not require frequent maintenance, (5) reproducible in the hands of different observers, (6) adaptable to different muscle groups, (7) portable so that it may be used in different settings, (8) fast, safe, comfortable, and inexpensive. The modified sphygmomanometer, as used to measure grip strength, can fulfill all the above requirements.

THE RHEUMATOLOGICAL PHYSICAL EXAMINATION
ISBN 0-8089-1824-9

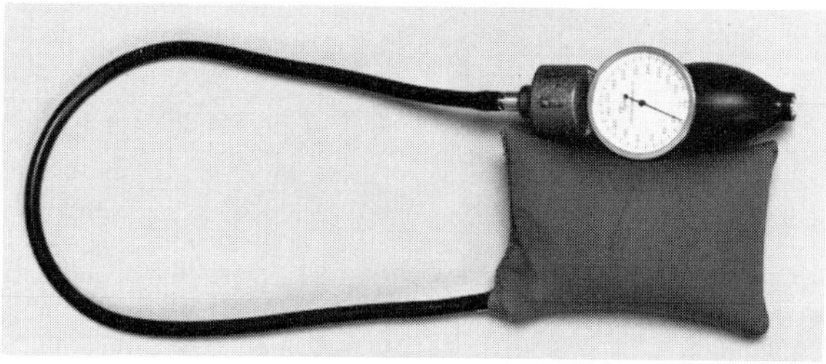

Figure 37

INSTRUMENT DESIGN

Figure 37. The modified sphygmomanometer.

The bladder of an aneroid sphygmomanometer is removed from its conventional cuff, folded into 3 equal sections and secured in a sewn cotton bag 12.5 cms. long, 9 cms. wide and 1.5 cms. thick.

MEASUREMENT TECHNIQUE

The bag is inflated to 100 mm Hg to remove the wrinkles in the bladder and then the pressure is reduced to a baseline of 20 mm Hg and the valve is closed tightly. This produces a measurement interval of 20–300 mm Hg.

The cuff is placed on the required lever point and the scale is positioned so that it can be seen by the examiner but not the examinee. The limb is adjusted to the starting position and the examinee is asked to hold that position. The examiner applies pressure gradually, increasing to a maximum over approximately 5 seconds. Pressure is applied by the flat of the hand, placed along the length of the cuff. The hand position is important. Gripping the cuff spuriously elevates the reading.

Muscle strength is the highest force recorded on the scale in mm Hg that the patient is able to sustain without movement. A fine muscle tremor may precede an abrupt cessation of muscle power. This tremor is accepted both as the end point of the test and as evidence that the patient is producing a maximal effort. If a tremor does not develop then the pressure required to produce movement at the joint is the measure of muscle strength.

It is most important that the cuff be placed on a specific point for each muscle group and the joint must be positioned at the same angle to obtain meaningful sequential studies.

Precautions

The measurement is valid only if it is painless. The patient must be cooperative and prepared to attempt a maximal contraction. The test objectives should be carefully explained and a trial run or demonstration should precede the test.

Limitations

The range of the instrument is from 20 mm Hg (baseline pressure in the cuff) to 300 mm Hg. Exceptional strength may exceed the scope of the instrument and the examiner must be strong enough to resist the patient's strength. This technique is not suitable for measuring muscles acting on the ankle, foot, wrist, or hand due to the small surfaces and the short lever arms.

Description of Technique by Muscle Group

The starting positions are selected to ensure patient safety and to improve effectiveness. Although the technique, as described, tests the muscle groups in one plane only, it can be adapted to test other planes and single muscles.

Hip Abduction (Figure 38.)

Starting position	Side lying
Lower leg	Fully flexed at hip and knee
Upper leg	Hip in neutral Knee extended
Position of cuff	Lengthwise on lateral side of thigh, just above the joint line of the knee. Patient resists against gravity.
Technique	Examiner presses on thigh downwards

Note—In stronger patients, the cuff may be placed above the lateral malleolus, provided there is no knee pathology on that side.

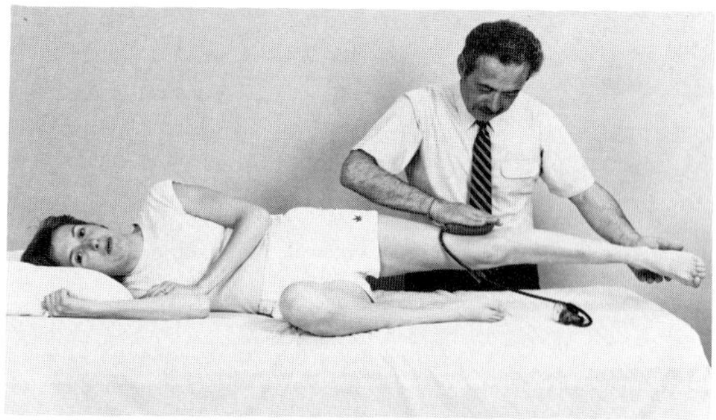

Figure 38

Hip Extension (Figure 39.)

Starting position	Side lying
Lower leg	Fully flexed at hip and knee
Upper leg	Hip neutral Knee extended
Position of Cuff	Lengthwise on posterior of thigh just above the joint line of the knee
Technique	Examiner presses on thigh forwards

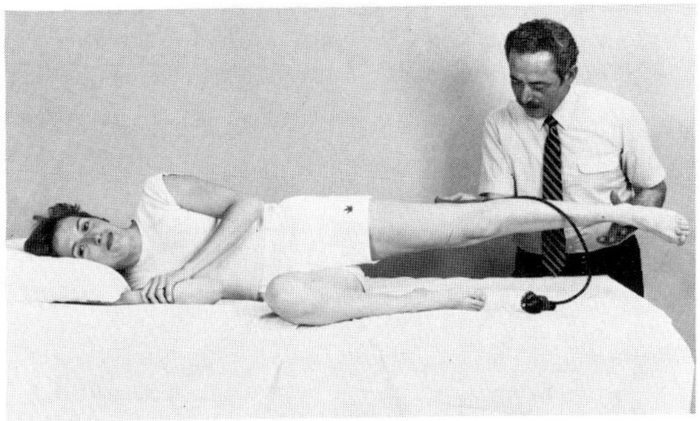

Figure 39

Knee Extension (Figure 40.)

Starting Position	Supine, arms at side
Tested leg	Supported on a quadriceps board with hip and knee flexed at 45 degrees
Position of Cuff	Anterior part of the leg, just above the ankle joint line
Technique	Examiner adjusts leg to 30 degrees flexion and presses downward

Note—a quadriceps board is seldom available. The sitting position, with the leg hanging is acceptable.

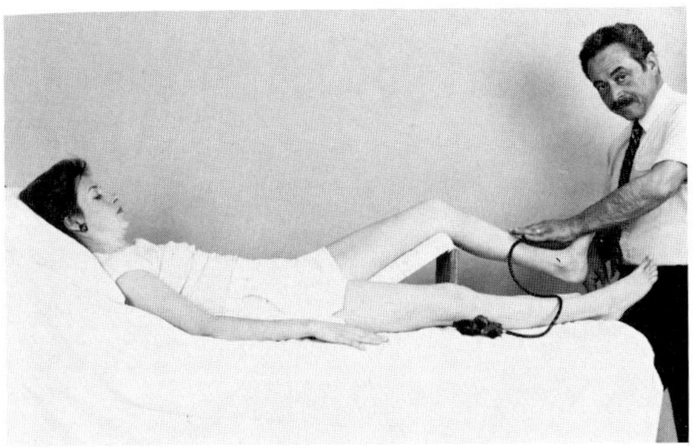

Figure 40

Knee Flexion (Figure 41.)

Starting Position	Prone, head resting on hands
Tested leg	Knee flexed at 30 degrees
Position of Cuff	At back of leg, longitudinally, just above the heel
Technique	Examiner presses downwards

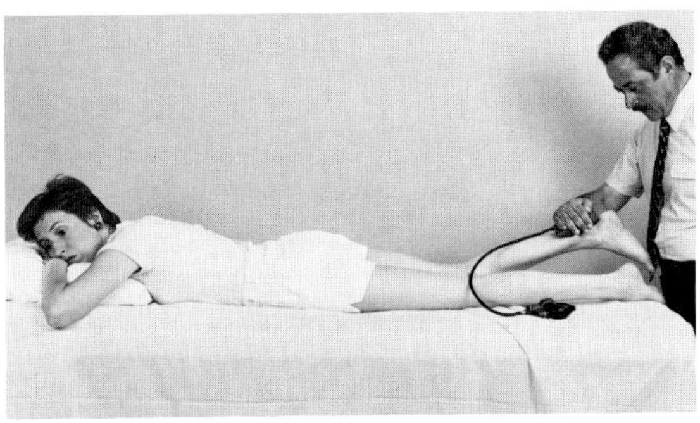

Figure 41

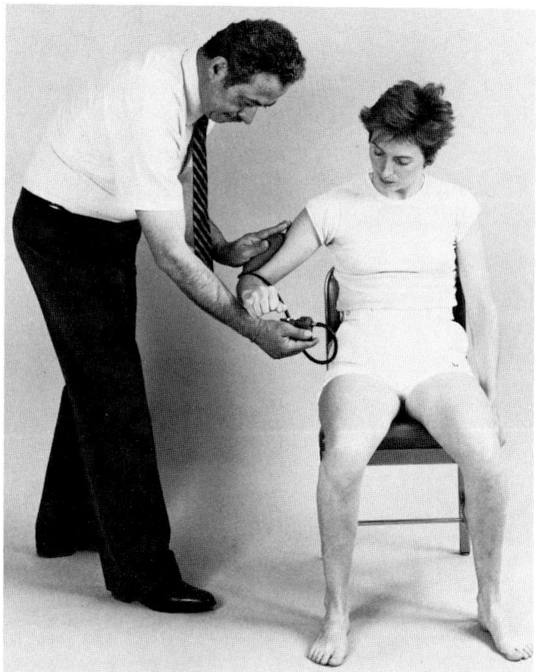

Figure 42

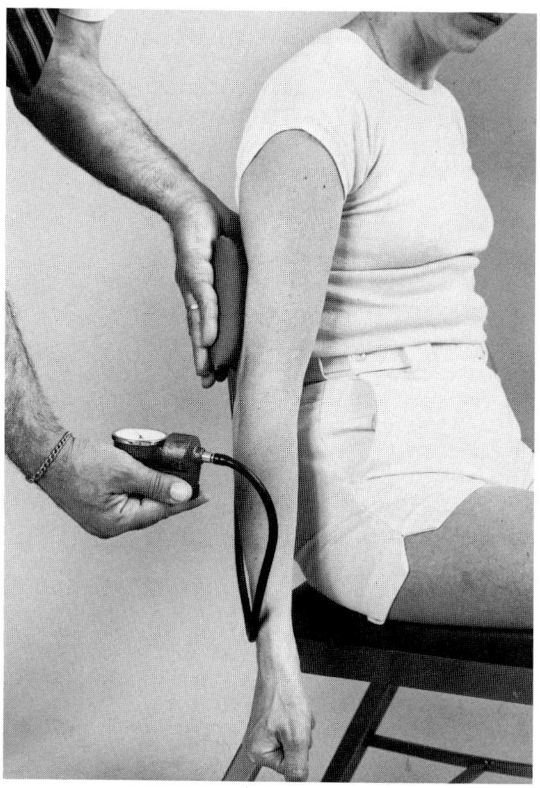

Figure 43

Shoulder Abduction (Figure 42.)

Starting Position	Sitting on a stable chair, back supported, heels pressed against front legs of the chair. One hand gripping edge of chair
Tested Arm	Held at 45 degrees abduction at the shoulder, elbow at 90 degrees of flexion
Position of Cuff	On lateral side of the arm, just above the lateral epicondyle
Technique	Examiner presses the arm downwards towards the body

Shoulder Extension (Figure 43.)

Starting Position	Sitting on a stable chair, back supported, heels pressed against the front legs of the chair, one hand gripping the edge of the chair
Tested arm	Held in 0 degrees of flexion at the shoulder
Position of Cuff	At the back of the arm, just above the olecranon
Technique	Examiner applies forward pressure

Shoulder Flexion (Figure 44.)

Starting Position — Sitting on a stable chair, back supported, heels pressed against the front legs of the chair, one hand gripping the edge of the chair.

Tested Arm — Held at 45 degrees forward flexion, elbow at 90 degrees

Position of Cuff — At the front of the arm, just above the elbow joint line.

Technique — Examiner applies downward pressure

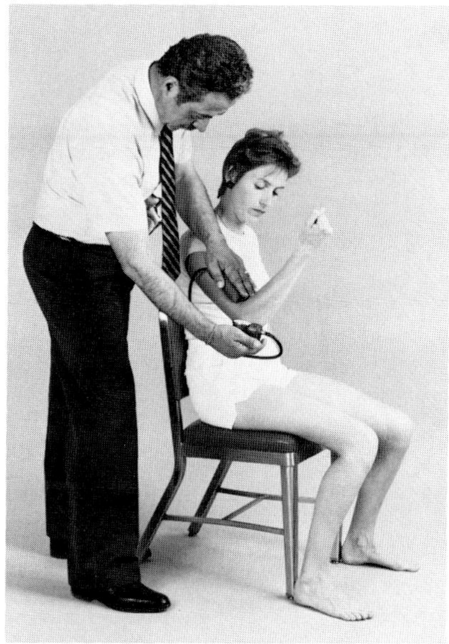

Figure 44

Elbow Flexion (Figure 45.)

Starting Position — Sitting on a stable chair, back supported, heels pressed against the front legs of the chair, one hand gripping the edge of the chair

Tested Arm — Held in 0 degrees flexion at the shoulder and 90 degrees flexion at the elbow, forearm supinated

Position of Cuff — On the anterior aspect of the forearm, just above the wrist joint line

Technique — Examiner presses downwards

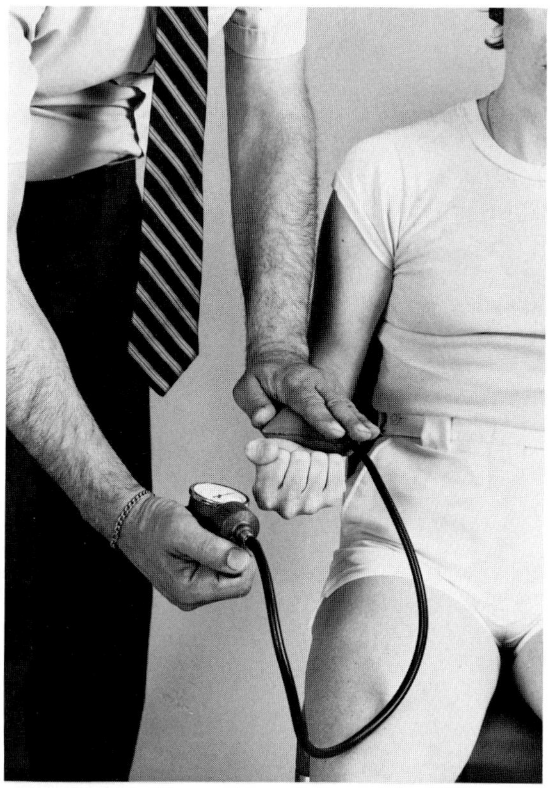

Figure 45

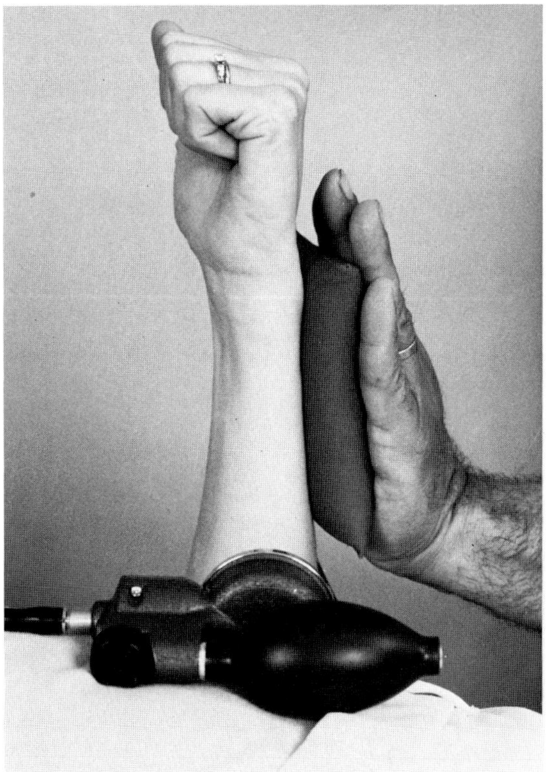

Figure 46

Elbow Extension (Figure 46.)

Starting Position	Lying on back, one arm by the side, hand gripping the edge of the plinth
Tested Arm	Held in 0 degrees flexion at the shoulder and 90 degrees of flexion at the elbow, forearm supinated
Position of Cuff	On the posterior aspect of the forearm, just above the wrist joint line
Technique	Examiner presses towards the patient's shoulder

Abdominal Muscles (Figure 47.)

Starting Position	Half lying, back supported 30 degrees from horizontal, hips and knees at 90 degrees of flexion, feet restrained by a belt or an assistant.
Test position	The patient is asked to sit up to 45 degrees from the horizontal
Position of Cuff	Across the sternum, level with the sternal notch
Technique	Examiner presses downward.

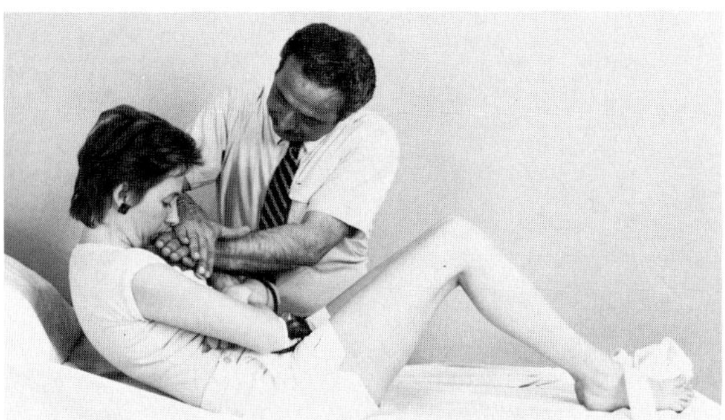

Figure 47

READING LIST

DEVELOPMENT

Moore KL: The Developing Human, Clinically Oriented Embryology. (ed 3). Philadelphia, WB Saunders Co, 1982.

Carter CO, Fairbanks TJ: The Genetics of Locomotor Disorders. London, Oxford University Press, 1974.

Williams PL, Warwick R: Gray's Anatomy (ed 36). Edinburgh, Churchill and Livingstone, 1982.

FUNCTIONAL ANATOMY

Kapandji IA: Physiology of the Joints (ed 5). Edinburgh, Churchill and Livingstone, 1980.

Wright V (Ed): Measurement of Joint Movement. Clinics in Rheumatic Diseases 8:3 1982.

Hollinshead WH, Jenkins DB, Functional Anatomy of the Limbs and Back (ed 5). Philadelphia, W.B. Saunders Co., 1981

Norkin CC, Levangie PK: Joint Structure and Function. Philadelphia, F.A. Davis Co., 1983

PHYSICAL EXAMINATION

Polley HF, Hunder GG: Rheumatological Interviewing and Physical Examination of the Joints (ed 2). Philadelphia, W.B. Saunders Co., 1978

Hoppenfeld S: Physical Examination of the Spine and Extremities, New York, Appleton-Century-Crofts, 1976

Apley AG, Solomon L: System of Orthopedics and Fractures (ed 6). London, Butterworth Scientific 1982

Fam A: M.S.K. Musculoskeletal Examination, Toronto, Collier Macmillan Co., 1980

REGIONAL REFERENCES

Friedman MH, Weisburg J, Agus B: Diagnosis and Treatment of Inflammation of the Temporomandibular Joint. Seminars in Rheumatic Disease 12, 1: Aug. 1982.

Guralnick W, Kaban LB, Merrill RG: Temporomandibular Joint Afflictions. New England Journal of Medicine 299:3, 1978

Lynch MA (ed): Burket's Oral Medicine (ed 7). Philadelphia, Lippincott, 1983.

Sweetman B: Development of the Spine and Biomechanics. in Low Back Pain, R. Grahame (ed). Annual Research Reviews. Eden Press, Churchill Livingstone, London 1979.

Roaf R: Spinal Deformities, London, Pitman Medical 1977

Keim H: The Adolescent Spine, New York, Springer-Verlag Co., 1976

Jackson R: The Cervical Syndrome (ed 4). Springfield Ill., Charles C Thomas, 1977.

Macnab I: Backache. Baltimore, Williams & Wilkins, 1977.

Hall H: Examination of the Patient with Low Back Pain. Bulletin on the Rheumatic Disease, 33:4 1983

Miller MH, Lee P, Smythe HA, Goldsmith CH: Measurement of Spinal Mobility in the Sagittal Plane. J Rheum., 11:4 1984

Bateman JE: The Shoulder and Neck. Philadelphia, W.B. Saunders Co., 1978

Caillet R: Shoulder Pain. Philadelphia, F.A. Davis Co., 1973

McCarthy SM, Ogden JA: Radiology of Post Natal Skeletal Development VI, Elbow Joint, Proximal Radius and Ulna. Skeletal Radiology 9:1 1982

Entin MA: Congenital Anomalies of the Hand. in Hand Surgery, J.E. Flynn (ed), Baltimore, Williams and Wilkins 1982

Flatt AE: Care of the Arthritic Hand (ed 4). Saint Louis, C.V. Mosby Co., 1983

Bellamy N, Rooney PJ: What do we know about the Sacroiliac Joint? Seminars in Rheumatic Disease, 12:3 1983

Moseley CF: Biomechanics of the Paediatric Hip, Orthopedic Clinics of North America 11:1 Jan 1980

Siffert RS: Patterns of Deformity of the Developing Hip. Clin. Orthop., 160: 1981

McDade W: Bow Legs and Knock Knees. Paed. Clin. North Am. 24:4 1977

Staheli LT: Torsional Deformity. Paed. Clin. North Am. 24:4 1977

Smillie IS: Diseases of the Knee Joint. Edinburgh, Churchill Livingstone 1980

Welsh RP: Knee Joint, Structure and Function. Clin. Orth. and Rel Res. 147:7-14, 1980.

Shybut GT, McGinty JB: The Office Evaluation of the Knee. Orthopedic Clinics of North America, 13:3 497-509, 1982.

Marshall JL, Baugher WH: Stability Examination of the Knee: A Simple Anatomical Approach. Clin Orthop and Rel Research. 78-83, 1982

Paulos L, Rusche K, Johnson C, Noyes FR: Patellar Malalignment: A Treatment Rationale. Physical Therapy 60:12 677-702, 1982.

Hughston JC, Andrews JR, Cross MJ, Moshi A: Classification of Knee Ligament Instabilities, Part 1 The Medial Compartment and Cruciate Ligaments, Part 2 The Lateral Compartment. J. Bone Joint Surg., 58A:2 1976

Fowler PJ: The Classification and Early Diagnosis of Knee Joint Instability. Clin Orthop and Rel Research 147: 15-21, 1980.

Coleman SH: Complex Foot Deformities in Children, Philadelphia, Lea and Febiger, 1983

Marrn RT (ed), DuVries' Surgery of the Foot, St Louis, C.V. Mosby Co., 1978

Inman VT: The Joints of the Ankle. Baltimore, Williams and Wilkins Co., 1976

Giannestras NJ: Foot Disorders: Medical and Surgical Management. (ed 2). Philadelphia, Lea and Febiger, 1973.

Inman VT: Human Locomotion. Canad. Med. Ass. J. 94: 1966

Kagen LJ: An Approach to the Patient with Myopathy, Bulletin on the Rheumatic Diseases 33;2, 1983.

Medical Research Council: Aids to the Investigation of Peripheral Nerve Injuries. War Memorandum No. 7, HMSO/ London, 1943.

Helewa A, Goldsmith CH, Smythe HA: The modified Sphyngomanometer—An instrument to measure muscle Strength: A validation Study. Journal of Chronic Diseases 34;7, 353-361 1981.

RHEUMATOLOGY TEXTS

McCarty DJ, (ed), Arthritis and Allied Conditions A Textbook of Rheumatology. Philadelphia, Lea and Febiger 1985

Kelley WN, Harris ED, Ruddy S, Sledge CB: Textbook of Rheumatology. Philadelphia, W.B. Saunders Co., 1985.

Index

Acetabulum, 105
Achilles tendon, 124
Achondroplasia, 34
Acromoiclavicular joint, 62
Anatomical snuff box, 86
Ankle, 124
Ankylosing spondylitis, 51
Apley's test, 120
Arthrogryposis multiplex congenita, 112

Baker's cyst, 116
Balloon sign, 35
Blount's disease, 112
Bones
- atlas, 45
- axis, 45
- calcaneus, 122
- capitate, 84
- clavicle, 61
- cuboid, 123
- cuneiform, 123
- femur, 105
- hamate, 84
- humerus, 66
- ilium, 105
- innominate, 102
- ischium, 105
- lunate, 84
- mandible, 39
- navicular, 122
- patella, 113
- pisiform, 84
- pubis, 105
- radius, 80
- sacrum, 103
- scaphoid, 84
- scapula, 61
- sesamoid, 113
- sternum, 62
- talus, 122
- tibia, 122
- trapezium, 84
- trapezoid, 84
- triquetrum, 84
- ulna, 80
- vertebra, 45
- zygomatic arch, 39

Boutonniere, 96
Brachydactyly, 92
Bunnell's test, 97

Calcaneus (ankle deformity), 122
Calcaneal spurs, 129
Capitulum, 74
Carpal height, 89
Carpal tunnel, 84
Carpometacarpal joint, 92
Cerebral palsy, 136
Cervical compression test, 50
Checklist, 36
Cleidocranial dysostosis, 60
Clubfoot, 122
Colles fracture, 87
Coracoclavicular bar, 60
Coracoid process, 61
Congenital dislocation of the hip, 106
Coronal plane, 30
Crepitus, 35
Crescent sign, 119
Cubitus valgus, 70
Cubitus varus, 70

DeQuervain's tenosynovitis, 89
Diabetes melitus, 136
Diarthrodial joints, 4
Diastomatomyelia, 44
Dinner fork deformity, 87
Dowager's hump, 51
Drawer sign, 119

Elbow, 73
Equinus, 122

Finger-fibula test, 56
Finklestein's test, 89

Gaenslen's test, 104
Gibbus, 51
Glenohumeral joint, 66
Glenoid, 66

Hallux valgus, 122
Hand, 91
Heelstrike, 134
Heel off, 135
Hemiplegia, 136
Hip, 105

Iliotibial band, 120
Initial contact, 134
Interphalangeal joints, 93
Intra-articular fibrocartilage, 6

Klippel Feil deformity, 44
Knee, 111
Knee-shoulder test, 104
Kyphosis, 30

Labrum, 6
Ligament
- annular, 74
- conoid, 62
- coracohumeral, 67
- cruciate, 115
- deltoid, 124
- flavum, 46
- glenohumeral, 67
- iliofemoral, 106
- inguinal, 109
- teres, 106
- transverse metacarpal, 93
- transverse metatarsal, 125
- trapezoid, 62
- triangular, 80
- spring, 123

Lister's tubercle, 86
Loading response, 134
Lobster claw, 92
Lordosis, 30
Lumbar spine, 55
Luschka (uncovertebral joints), 43

Marfan's syndrome, 31
McMurray's Test, 120
Meckel's cartilage, 38
Median nerve, 89
Medical Research Council, 139
Megalodactyly, 92
Meningomyelocoele, 44
Meniscus, 113
Metacarpophalangeal joints, 93
Metatarsal compression test, 129
Metatarsophalangeal joints, 125
Metatarsus varus, 122
Midstance, 135
Midtarsal joint, 125
Mirror hands, 92
Morquio's syndrome, 44
Mons pubis, 104
Muscular dystrophy, 136
Muscles
- abductor pollicis longus, 85
- adductor magnus, 106
- biceps, 75
- biceps femoris, 106
- brachialis, 75
- brachioradialis, 75
- deltoid, 67
- extensor carpi radialis, 85
- extensor carpi ulnaris, 85
- extensor hallucis longus, 124
- extensor indicis, 85
- extensor pollicis longus, 85
- flexor carpi ulnaris, 85
- flexor carpi radialis, 85
- gastrocnemius, 124
- gluteus maximus, medius, 106
- gracilis, 115
- iliopsoas, 106
- infraspinatus, 67
- latissimus dorsi, 67
- levator scapulae, 62
- masseter, 39
- obturator, 106
- palmaris longus, 85
- pectineus, 106
- pectoralis major, 67
- pectoralis minor, 62
- peroneus brevis, longus, 124
- piriformis, 106
- pterygoid, 39
- quadriceps, 115
- rectus femoris, 106
- rhomboids, 62
- sartorius, 115
- semimembranosis, 115
- semitendinosis, 115
- serratus anterior, 62
- subscapularis, 62
- supinator, 81
- supraspinatus, 67
- temporalis, 39
- tensor fascia latae, 106
- teres minor, 67
- tibialis anterior, 124
- tibialis posterior, 124
- trapezius, 62
- triceps, 75

Neck, 43
Notocord, 43

Occipital axis, 54
Odontoid, 45
Olecranon, 74
Osteophyte, 32

Palmar fascia, 94
Palm up position, 70
Parotid gland, 40
Patellar apprehension test, 120
Patellar tap, 118
Pes cavus, 122
Pes planus, 122
Phalen's test, 89
Piano key sign, 82
Pierre Robin syndrome, 38
Pivot shift, 120
Plantar fascia, 123
Polydactyly, 92
Polyphalagy, 92
Protrusio acetabuli, 106
Push off, 134

Radial nerve, 81
Radioulnar joints, 79
Radioulnar synostosis, 79
Rickets, 112
Rotoscoliosis, 51

Sacciform recess, 80
Sacrococcygeal joint, 57
Sacroiliac joint, 101
Sagittal plane, 30
Scoliosis, 30
Shoulder, 65
Shoulder girdle, 59
Sphyngomanometer, 139
Spinal stenosis, 44
Spondyloepiphyseal dysplasia, 44
Spondylolisthesis, 31
Sprengel's deformity, 59
Shober test, 56
Slocum test, 120
Square shoulder, 69
Sternoclavicular joint, 62
Subtalar joint, 125
Surface tension, 6
Swan neck deformity, 96
Syndactyly, 92
Symphysis, 3

Tabes dorsalis, 136
Talipes, 122

Temperomandibular joint, 37
Tender points, 54
Terminal swing, 135
Thomas test, 110
Tibial torsion, 117
Tinel's sign, 89
Toe deformities, 127
Trendelenberg test, 110
Triangle sign, 77
Trigger finger, 97
Trochanteric bursitis, 109
Tuck sign, 89
Turner's syndrome, 73

Uncovertebral joints (of Luschka), 45
Ulnar nerve, 77

Z deformity, 96